EAT
TO
COMPETE

GW00937852

EAT
TO
COMPETE

sports excellence
through good nutrition

JENI PEARCE

REED

Published by Reed Books, a division of Octopus Publishing Group (NZ) Ltd,
39 Rawene Road, Birkenhead, Auckland. Associated companies, branches
and representatives throughout the world.

This book is copyright. Except for the purpose of fair reviewing, no part of this
publication may be reproduced or transmitted in any form or by any means,
electronic or mechanical, including photocopying, recording, or any information
storage and retrieval system, without permission in writing from the publisher.
Infringers of copyright render themselves liable to prosecution.

ISBN 0 7900 0087 3

© Jeni Pearce 1990

First published 1990
Reprinted 1990, 1991, 1992, 1993

Designed by Graeme Leather
Typeset by Sabagraphics
Printed by South Wind Production, Singapore

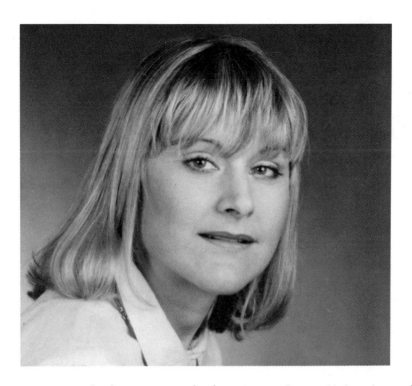

Jeni Pearce studied nutrition and education at Otago University and pursued her interest in education at Auckland Secondary Teachers' College. She gained her postgraduate training as a dietitian at Christchurch Hospital. After further hospital experience she went to Iowa State University to complete a master of science degree in nutrition education.

Based in the Auckland/Waikato area, Jeni currently runs a private practice as a Consultant Dietitian and Sports Nutritionist in Hamilton. She conducts a number of clinics in the Waikato and has held seminars on nutrition-related topics throughout New Zealand. In addition, she lectures regularly on sports nutrition at Waikato Polytechnic.

Jeni is nutrition adviser to the Commonwealth Games catering committee. Among the individual sporting personalities she has advised are Sandra Mallett, John Kirwan and Tracey Fear. She has planned nutritional programmes for the New Zealand netball team, the junior and senior rowing teams and the junior and senior women's squash teams, as well as triathletes, bodybuilders, boxers, marathon runners, rugby league players and cricketers. She has also advised aerobics instructors and coaches, and brings to her writing the practical experience of working with a wide range of sports participants — from children and those with special needs to competitive athletes and veterans.

Acknowledgements

My thanks go to the editorial team at Heinemann Reed and to Bob Carter, who provided the photographs. I would like to express my special gratitude and appreciation to the many New Zealand athletes who gave me the motivation to write this book and who helped at various stages of its preparation.

Contents

Introduction

There are no magic foods for enhancing performance in sport, but poor nutrition can prevent athletes from achieving their potential and hinder performance and endurance. Good nutrition will not create a champion overnight but it may help reduce the time of an event by a few crucial seconds or allow an athlete to run a few extra kilometres, to maintain, increase or reduce body weight, to lift that extra kilogram, or to produce that final last minute effort that wins the game. Sports performance improves with wise and balanced nutrition and crumbles with nutritional deficiencies, imbalances and fads.

Eat to Compete examines the relationship between sound nutrition, body composition, weight control and exercise performance. The relationship between each of these factors, as well as their individual importance in sports performance and good health, is illustrated.

Good nutrition is essential for growth and development but is often only considered by the coach, trainer, athlete or player briefly during the season, if at all. For effective performance, good nutrition is critical at all times — pre-season, during the season and off-season. Practising good nutritional habits should be part of the total lifestyle and training programmes for all sportsmen and sportswomen. The principles that apply to body weight control and sound nutrition also apply to the non-sportsperson. An athlete or sportsperson may be concerned with gaining muscle mass (or fat-free weight) and the non-active person may wish to avoid obesity and the problems associated with this condition. The procedure for achieving both these goals is similar.

Good performance doesn't just happen. A sound knowledge of

1

a number of factors — such as coaching, training, discipline and genetics — is necessary. Good nutrition is one of these important factors, yet it is often the least understood and the least applied.

The higher the level, the more competitive an event, the faster the opposition, the greater the degree of skill — the more important is the individual sportsperson's nutritional state. When winning depends on a split second, a few millimetres, a last minute sprint or the final stage of an endurance event, good nutrition can make the difference.

Participation in sport in New Zealand has increased dramatically and more New Zealanders than ever now compete internationally. Our increasing participation in Olympic and Commonwealth Games has highlighted the involvement of exercise in our lives. Exercise and the role of nutrition is relevant for the casual participant who competes for fun and enjoyment as well as the serious competitive sportsperson. There are several recommendations that, when followed, can enable people to get more out of their sport. Benefits include improving times, endurance, speed, concentration and enjoyment. No one would put inferior petrol or oil in their car, yet many people fuel their bodies with inadequate, unbalanced or inappropriate food and expect top performance.

What do you know about the science of shaping up for good nutrition? Read each of the following statements and note whether it is true or false:

- To cope with the stress of training and conditioning you will need some form of vitamin/mineral supplementation. T F

- To lose a few pounds quickly it is a good idea to stop eating for a time and train harder. T F

- If you drink more than a swallow of fluid before you exercise or run, or if you stop running and satisfy your thirst, you risk painful cramps. T F

- The effect of exercise on maintaining or building muscular fitness does not occur until you have reached fatigue. T F

- If you have a tendency to perspire freely on hot days you should take a salt tablet when you exercise. T F

- One way to become fit through good nutrition is to cut as much sugar and starch out of your diet as possible. T F

- About 40 minutes of running daily will burn calories but will also increase appetite. T F

- If you run, swim or perform vigorous activity your body needs extra protein for energy and to build muscle. T F

2

- Sportspeople who have a lean body frame, irrespective of their particular activity, do not need to consider the fat content of their diet. T F

- Honey, a high energy source, is absorbed faster into the blood, is healthier and contains fewer calories than sugar. T F

- Following a diet without red meat places sportspeople at risk of developing severe nutritional deficiencies. T F

- To obtain a competitive edge, athletes, especially runners, must maintain a very low body weight because the lower the body weight and body fat levels the faster their race time. T F

All these are false. The truth about these factors will be found throughout the following chapters.

The perfect state of nutrition is not achieved by any last-minute tactics, such as the pre-event meal or a few days on a special diet just before an event, race or game. It is the care and attention applied to long-term eating patterns that makes the difference.

There are five stages where good nutrition and what you eat play a critical role in your health, well-being and sports performance. These are:

Baseline eating patterns What you eat every day. These are foods for good general health for everyone.

Training meals Which foods need increasing. Special consideration must be given to increased energy intake, eating difficulties caused by the demands of training schedules, weight gain and weight loss.

Pre-competition foods Special considerations are needed in meal planning for endurance events and to provide appropriate carbo-hydrate loading.

Food for competition What to eat for top performance on the day. Things to consider include the weather, level of activity, multi events, competition timetables, eating out and special issues related to travel and takeaways.

Eating for recovery Which foods aid recovery and what to do if appetite diminishes. This includes off-season eating patterns.

While there is no magic food or group of foods that will cover in-adequacies in training or ability, an individual's knowledge and practice of good nutrition can provide a competitive edge and help determine a winner.

The baseline eating pattern involves examining the foods eaten daily and the overall eating patterns. This is the type of eating pattern that should be followed by all New Zealanders at all ages, activity levels and lifestyles — not just sportsmen and sportswomen. Owing to a higher energy expenditure the athlete or sportsperson's total kilojoule intake is generally higher than sedentary individuals'. Requirements do, however, vary according to body size, sex, age, sport and level of training.

The national diet survey in 1977 reported that New Zealand adults increased in weight an average of 5 kg between their 20s and 40s. Energy intakes were higher than for most other developed countries. Protein and cholesterol intakes (cholesterol intakes averaged 500–700 mg/day for men and 300–400 mg/day for women) were high and fat made up 41 percent of the energy.

Nutritional problems affect the general health of all New Zealanders, both active and non-active. These problems can relate to heart disease, obesity, diabetes, cancer and high blood pressure. As well as being a health problem, obesity is a leading cause of inactivity. Overweight individuals must expend more energy simply to move about and this movement causes an increase in the heart rate. New Zealanders continue to eat a diet that is high in salt, fat, sugar and alcohol and low in fibre and complex carbohydrates. Sportspeople, in particular, need to be encouraged to select a balanced diet from the wide range of foods available to them. This improves health and well-being and may result in improved endurance and performance.

The point of reference used in this book is the *Nutritional Guidelines for New Zealanders*. This is a set of recommendations designed to improve our general health. Regardless of whether you participate in a particular sport, following these guidelines will establish a solid nutritional foundation. There are seven basic guidelines: eat a variety of foods; maintain weight within a reasonable range; don't eat too much sugar; eat adequate dietary fibre; don't eat too much salt; don't drink too much alcohol; and don't eat too much fat.

These have been expanded into 10 guidelines, to include information particularly important for the sportsperson. The nutritional guidelines for active New Zealanders are:

Choose a wide selection of foods.

Eat adequate carbohydrate.

Keep body weight within a reasonable range.

Use less sugar.

Eat less fat, especially saturated fat.

Ensure an adequate intake of protein.

Take care with salt.

Drink sufficient fluid and use alcohol in moderation.

Eat adequate fibre.

Vitamin, mineral and protein supplements are not recommended for general use — take them only if special circumstances apply.

Several studies analysing the diet of sportspeople report similar observations. Many athletes fail to reach the recommended intake of carbohydrate. Intakes of protein are often far above the recommended level and there is no need to take additional protein. Fat intakes vary among different groups. However, many sports enthusiasts consume above 35 percent of their energy input from fat sources. Recreational runners consume higher intakes of energy from protein, fat and alcohol and less from carbohydrate than marathon and endurance athletes. Iron and calcium intakes are a concern for active women and endurance runners.

The following chapters examine each of the 10 recommendations for active people in more detail. Information on individual sports, women, children, veterans and vegetarian eating patterns is presented in later chapters.

It should be noted that food information tables in this book, where unsourced, are based on figures provided by the DSIR's *New Zealand Food Composition Tables*, Palmerston North, 1989, and the Australian Government's *Metric Tables of Composition of Australian Food*. Local data has been used wherever possible.

1
Baseline eating patterns

Training, genetics and determination all play a role in athletic performance. Nutrition is the next most important consideration for an athlete or any person participating seriously in sport. The aim of sports nutrition is to optimise performance to achieve a competitive edge while maintaining an interest in meals. Good baseline eating patterns fuel the body with energy for hard training sessions and peak performance. Poor nutrition weakens the potential of the sport participant by reducing the energy available for exercise or supplying an imbalance or inadequate range of various nutrients essential for energy release.

If you are exercising on a regular basis you are on the way to becoming fit. Exercise and eating right form the basis of a healthy lifestyle. A good eating programme or food plan should not consist of self-denial, restrictions or unappetising meals. Eating a wide variety of food is important for all sportspeople in order that they retain interest in the food being eaten, but also to ensure all the nutrients essential to good health and performance are consumed. The body requires about 40 different nutrients to stay healthy. There is no perfect food that will supply all the nutrients needed by the body for good health. One food that comes close is breast milk. It provides adequate levels of most nutrients for infants in the first six months of life, and the infant has additional stores of iron at birth to carry it through the first six months or so until solids are introduced.

Eating only one food (for example, only bananas, bread or grape-fruit) increases the risk of essential nutrients being excluded from the body. If this type of eating behaviour continues over a long period of time the risk of developing nutritional deficiencies increases. In addition, this diet soon becomes uninteresting and boredom results.

In order to achieve the nutritional goal of eating a wide variety of food choose food based on the healthy food pyramid.

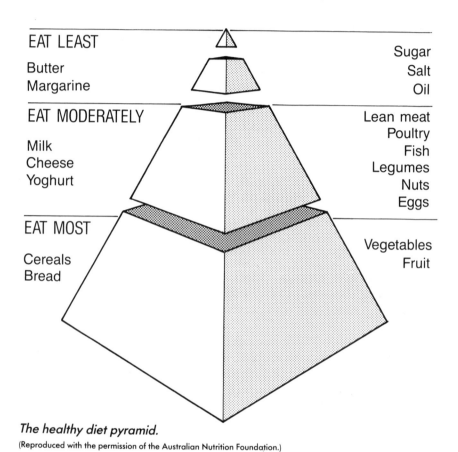

EAT LEAST
Butter
Margarine

Sugar
Salt
Oil

EAT MODERATELY
Milk
Cheese
Yoghurt

Lean meat
Poultry
Fish
Legumes
Nuts
Eggs

EAT MOST
Cereals
Bread

Vegetables
Fruit

The healthy diet pyramid.
(Reproduced with the permission of the Australian Nutrition Foundation.)

Eat more from the fruit, vegetable, bread and cereal (especially the wholegrain varieties) food groups. This will provide energy from carbohydrate sources, to allow for training and general exercise as well as competitive games and events. When the energy level provided by any particular eating pattern is too low to meet the needs of a sportsperson, fatigue occurs earlier and performance diminishes.

Choose moderate servings of milk, cheese, eggs, yoghurt, meat, poultry, legumes (dried peas, beans, lentils) and nuts. These foods tend to be higher in hidden fats and oils so trim off all excess fat or choose the lower fat variety. Eat only small amounts of butter,

7

margarine, oil, salt and sugar. These foods are low nutrient density foods. They provide a high proportion of kilojoules and little else in the way of nutrients.

The food groups

Foods can be divided into five main groups as follows:

Milk and milk products   Protein, calcium, riboflavin, vitamins A and D are provided by food from this food group.

Fruit and vegetables   Foods from this food group are excellent sources of vitamins A and C, minerals and carbohydrate and are also low in fat.

Bread and cereals   Fibre, carbohydrate and B vitamins are well provided through the selection of foods from this food group.

Meat and alternatives   Meat, fish, poultry, legumes, nuts and seeds. These foods are good sources of protein, some minerals and most B vitamins.

Fats, sweets and alcohol   These foods are high in energy content and are only required in very small amounts. Some useful amounts of vitamins A and D are also provided.

By eating some food from each of the first four food groups — bread and cereals; fruit and vegetables; milk and milk products; meat and alternatives (dried beans and lentils) — each day, a balanced eating pattern can be achieved in the long term.

Sportspeople require a sound knowledge of the principles of good nutrition and must know how to select a variety of foods from the food pyramid and basic food groups. When energy needs are met and the recommended nutrients are consumed vitamin and mineral supplements should not be necessary. Exceeding the requirements for good health does not enhance performance and in some specific cases could be detrimental to health and performance.

The following lists indicate how much you can eat of different foods to get enough of the nutrients without too much fat, sugar or salt.

Eat as much as you like from:
    vegetables (without added butter, fat or oil);
    fresh fruit;
    salad vegetables (easy on the dressing);
    cottage cheese;

white fish (steamed or baked, not fried);
natural unsweetened yoghurt.

Eat in moderation from:
lean red meat, trim pork and lean lamb;
white meat — chicken and turkey;
low fat cheeses;
eggs;
milk (choose the low fat variety);
sardines, salmon, tuna and shellfish;
bread and pasta;
rice and potatoes;
legumes and dried beans;
dried, baked, stewed and canned fruit;
ice cream;
cereals (especially whole grains, but take care with sweetened cereals — for example, Honey Puffs);
nuts;
unsweetened fruit juices.

Eat only a little from:
butter, margarine, oil and lard;
fried foods;
sugar, sweets and chocolate;
jam, honey, marmalade, syrups and treacle;
salty snacks (peanuts and chips);
fatty meats — sausages, meat pies and mince;
pastry;
biscuits and rich cakes;
sweet drinks, including sweet soda drinks.

Nutrient content of foods

The amounts to be eaten from each of the five main food groups vary with individual age, activity, body weight and overall health, but selecting a variety of foods from within each food group is important. It is essential to avoid relying on only a few favourite foods. Try small servings of unfamiliar foods.

Milk and milk products

Milk has been a valuable contributor to the New Zealand diet for a number of years. Recent advances in packaging and marketing have made a wider choice of milk and milk products available to the consumer. More lower fat varieties now line supermarket shelves.

Foods included in this food group are: milk (whole, homogenised, 2-Ten, fat reduced, low fat, trim, skim, dried, long life, evaporated and condensed), cheese, cottage cheese, yoghurt, and any products made with milk. These foods are excellent sources of calcium, are high in protein and riboflavin (B_2), contain vitamin B_{12} and some vitamins A and D.

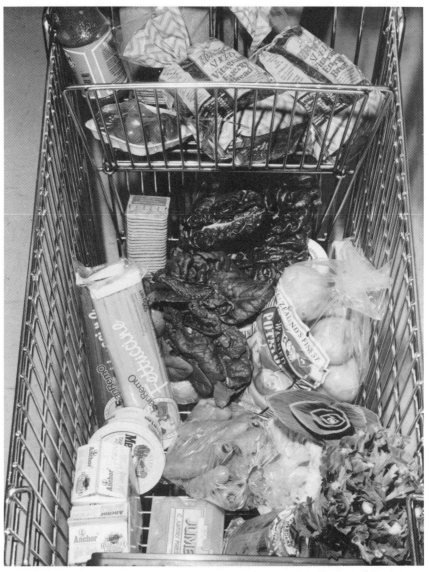

A healthy selection of foods based on the food groups fills this trolley.

Variations in the nutrient content among the diferent milks now determine their use by the sportsperson. These variations include energy value, percentage fat, level of fat soluble vitamins, protein, calcium and carbohydrate. For example, trim milk contains more calcium, less fat and has a lower energy value than homogenised milk. As the flavouring in flavoured milk contains more sugar the carbohydrate level and energy value of this milk is higher. Much of the fat of whole milk is removed to provide skim or trim milk (from around 4.2 percent to 0.5 percent fat content). With the removal of fat the fat-soluble vitamins and energy content of the milk are also reduced. The energy value of skim milk is almost half that found in whole milk. This is the reason behind the label 'not suitable as a complete milk food for infants' found on skim and trim milks.

■ NUTRIENT CONTENT OF MILK PER 100 ML

Milk	CHO* g	Fat g	Prot g	Calcium mg	Energy kJ/Cal
Flavoured	8.5	2.0	3.3	140	275/65
Whole	4.7	4.2	3.4	120	293/70
Homogenised	4.7	3.3	3.4	120	260/62
2-Ten (fat reduced)	5.5	2.0	4.0	140	236/56
Trim	5.5	0.5	4.4	160	188/45
Skim	5.0	0.1	3.8	123	151/35

*CHO = carbohydrate
(Source: NZ Dairy Company — Fluid Milk Division.)

■ ■ ■

Choose the lower fat varieties such as skim or trim milk (remember these are not suitable for infants and young children), low fat cheeses, and yoghurt, particularly if weight reduction is needed. If you do not use milk products then extra care will be needed to obtain an adequate amount of calcium. At least two servings from this group are required per day.

Fruit and vegetables

These foods are high in vitamins (especially vitamins A and C), minerals and fibre and can also be valuable sources of energy without increasing the fat content of a meal. At least four or more servings should be eaten from this food group each day — raw, cooked, steamed, boiled, microwaved, fresh, frozen or canned. Watch the salt level of canned vegetables. Use fresh vegetables and fruits where possible. Some frozen varieties may contain a higher nutrient content of various vitamins when compared to 'fresh' vegetables that have been displayed in retail outlets for some time.

Fruits contain a high water content (ranging from 70 to 90 percent), contain carbohydrate, particularly bananas and avocados, and provide a valuable source of dietary fibre. They are low in protein and fat (excluding avocados and olives which contain a higher fat content than most other fruits). To assist with keeping the fat content low, roast or fry vegetables only for special occasions. The fat added to potatoes and other vegetables increases the calorie content, which has resulted in people limiting the choice of these foods. Potatoes provide valuable contributions to a meal, supplying vitamin C, thiamine and iron. Use small amounts of iodised salt in the cooking.

High concentrations of nutrients are supplied through the inclusion of dark green leafy vegetables in the food plan. Generally they are excellent sources of fibre, vitamin C (eaten fresh or with minimal heat), carotene (vegetable source of vitamin A), riboflavin, folic acid, iron and calcium. Small amounts of B_1, B_3 and vitamin E are also available. However, these values are susceptible to change due to soil composition, harvesting methods, storage, processing and cooking methods.

■ VITAMIN C CONTENT

Food	Serving	Vitamin C mg
Apple	1 average (80 g)	6.5
Banana	1 average (100 g)	10.0
Kiwifruit	2 medium (100 g)	100.0
Orange	1 average (85 g)	43.0
Fruit juice	1 glass (250 ml)	88.0
Cabbage	1 cup raw	28.0
Cabbage	1 cup cooked	10.0
Carrots	½ cup	5.0
Peas	½ cup frozen	16.0
Potato	½ cup	14.0

■ ■ ■

Fruits and vegetables can be divided into two further groups based on the amount of kilojoules (energy) they provide in the form of carbohydrate. There is a group of fruits and vegetables that provide bulk and are very low in energy content (lettuce, cabbage) and another group that is somewhat higher (kumara, yams). Obtaining a balance between these two groups can be an effective method of weight control, achieving a balanced diet or increasing the energy content of an eating plan without added fat.

It is important for any athlete or person actively involved in sport to eat a wide variety of fruit and vegetables regularly. These foods provide excellent sources of carbohydrates and are very low in fat, so they are ideal fuel for sport.

■ *FRUIT AND VEGETABLES CONTAINING HIGHER ENERGY VALUES*

Fruit	Vegetables
Apples	Beetroot
Bananas	Broad beans
Dried fruit	Coconuts
Canned fruit	Carrots (large serving)
Grapes	Cassava
Oranges	Corn
Pears	Kumara
Peaches	Mixed vegetables
Pineapples	Parsnips
All berry fruit	Peas
Avocado*	Potatoes
Stewed fruit	Pumpkin/squash
Tropical fruit	Taro
	Yams/sweet potatoes

*High fat content

■ ■ ■

For athletes at ideal body weight all fruit and vegetables may be eaten freely. However, for those wishing to reduce weight these are fruit and vegetables that may be eaten freely:

Fruit Unsweetened rhubarb, passionfruit, tamarillos, watermelon (small serving), melons, small grapefruit, lemons, limes and pepino.

Vegetables All other vegetables not listed, especially green leafy vegetables such as lettuce, asparagus, silverbeet; cabbage, peppers, spinach, beans (including beansprouts), mushrooms, onions, cauliflower, watercress and swede.

It is important to have some foods from each group at meal times. For weight control try to keep a balance between the energy content of these foods. To increase weight add more of the higher energy vegetables and fruits into the eating plan. For weight reduction try to include at least two of the higher energy vegetables in the evening meal and choose more from the other group. Rice and pasta may be substituted for one of the higher energy vegetables.

Bread and cereals

This food group includes: flour (white and wholemeal), wheat, rice, pasta (spaghetti, macaroni, noodles), oats, barley and rye, breakfast cereals and all other cereals. The bread and cereal group supplies energy, carbohydrate and protein in the greatest quantities.

The cereal foods (especially rice, wheat and corn) are the staple food sources for many different population groups throughout the world. Wheat is the predominant cereal in New Zealand. Most cereals contain 10-12 percent protein (with the exception of rice at 8 percent) and provide up to 70 percent of the energy in the diet in many parts of the world, particularly in the developing countries. Carbohydrate, which supplies this proportion of energy in the diet, is ideal for sportspeople in heavy endurance training.

For New Zealanders, who usually obtain 40 percent of their energy from cereals (carbohydrates), the recommendation is to increase this food group, especially the high fibre foods. With an increase in the bread and cereal foods it is important to ensure that the fats (butter and margarine) and sweets (sugar, jam, marmalade and honey) are not also increased. Other nutrients supplied by the bread and cereal group include vitamin B, especially thiamine (B_1) and niacin (B_2); vitamin E, various minerals (magnesium, potassium, phosphate and calcium) and trace elements (iron, zinc, copper and manganese). Cereals generally are inadequate sources of vitamin A (except for maize and corn products), vitamin C and vitamin D.

On bread labels, ash is often listed under the nutrient contents. This refers to a measurement of the minerals present. Take care when purchasing cereal foods because salt and sugar (such as honey, glucose, malt or sucrose) are often added, either as preservatives or flavouring agents.

The carbohydrate content of bread and cereals is called starch and is broken down by the body's digestive process (using many enzymes) into simpler substances, including glucose, which are absorbed into the bloodstream.

The extraction rate of New Zealand flour (78 percent) is higher than in other developed countries (70-72 percent). This means more of the bran and germ layers are retained in the flour, so it is not necessary to fortify New Zealand flour as is done in other countries.

There have been changes in the purchasing patterns of bread in recent times. A study in 1978 indicated 90 percent preference for white bread. In 1983 this had dropped to 70 percent and to 60 percent by 1985. Whole grains are preferable as foods made from unrefined cereals contain a higher concentration of protein, B vitamins, minerals and dietary fibre. Four or more servings from this food group can be eaten daily.

■ NUTRIENT CONTENT OF CEREALS PER 100 GRAMS

Cereal	Protein g	CHO‡ g	B_1 μg	B_3 mg
White flour	11	75	270	1.6
Wholegrain flour	13	66	460	5.6
Baking bran	14	27	890	29.6
Puffed wheat	12	66	*	4.7
Rolled oats	12	73	500	1.0
Weetbix	11	70	*	1.5
White bread	8	46	120	0.9
Wholegrain bread †	8	30	275	3.0
Cornflakes	9	85	*	0.03
Muesli	7	62	30	2.6
Rice bubbles	6	88	*	0.07

*New Zealand value not presently available
†Average values of five leading brands
‡Carbohydrate
(Data adapted from Gillies & Swindells, *Today's Foods — Tomorrow's Health*.)

■ ■ ■

Meat and alternatives

The energy value of meat varies depending on its fat content. These foods are excellent sources of protein, niacin (vitamin B_3), vitamins B_6 and B_{12}, iron, phosphorus, zinc and riboflavin (B_2). Useful amounts of vitamin A and D, copper, selenium and magnesium are also provided. Meat, however, is a poor source of carbohydrates and vitamins C and E, and can be high in saturated fat. Though many forms of offal (such as liver, kidney, tongue and sweetbreads) are high in cholesterol, these foods are concentrated sources of vitamins and minerals (iron, zinc, copper and selenium). Used occasionally, they make a useful contribution to the diet. Marine fish provide useful amounts of iodine, selenium and fluoride, and whole fish eaten with bones (tuna, salmon and sardines) contain valuable supplies of calcium.

Meat, particularly red meat, is an important part of our culture and the central feature of the main meal for many New Zealanders. The abundance of meat and dairy products available in New Zealand has contributed to a high intake of protein and fat. The recommendation for meat is to choose the low fat variety and take care with the size of servings. Cut all the fat off the meat before and after cooking, grill rather than fry and eat a smaller portion. Remove the skin from chicken and include more white flesh meat into meal plans (for example, fish, chicken and turkey). However, to help maintain iron levels it is helpful to include red meat in eating patterns. Meat also supplies most of the dietary vitamin B_{12}.

Vegetarians must take extra care to include particular vegetables, especially the green-leaf varieties, to obtain adequate folic acid and iron. With the reduction in meat intake it is also important to obtain an adequate supply of protein from other sources. Alternatives include dried beans, peas and lentils. These foods are often referred to as pulses or legumes and are a central feature in the vegetarian diet. Examples include lima beans, soya beans, haricot beans, chick peas and split peas. These foods are high in protein and many are also high in fat and provide carbohydrates. Nuts and seeds are popular additions to muesli and salads, or can be eaten as snacks. Their high energy value is provided by the unsaturated oil they contain. However, as coconut oil contains saturated fats its use should be limited.

At least one serving of food from this food group should be included in the daily intake, but take care to avoid excessive fat consumption. Valuable contributions to nutritional status are made through consuming moderate servings of these foods.

Fat, sweets and alcohol
The eating patterns of many New Zealanders include more servings from this food group than is desirable for good health. This leads to a diet that is high in fat, high in sugar and contains an excessive energy intake. Foods in this group include butter, Chefade, margarine, oils, potato chips and other fried snacks, cream, chocolate, salad dressings and mayonnaise. The sweets include sugar (all varieties from brown, raw and white to icing sugar and sugar cubes), golden syrup, sweet jelly, lollies, sweet syrups such as treacle, pancake syrup, jam, honey and marmalade. This food group also includes all forms of alcohol.

These foods contain the greatest source of energy weight for weight when compared with other foods. The fat group provides vitamins A, D, E and K; essential fatty acids; cholesterol; and energy. All of these nutrients are essential for important body functions. Therefore, total exclusion of fat from the regular eating pattern can be hazardous to health. It is the proportion of these foods in the baseline eating plan that is relevant. Keep the use of these foods to a minimum.

The present intake of fat in the New Zealand diet is around 40 percent, which is higher than the intake in Australia (35 percent). The recommended level of fat intake for the New Zealand diet is 30–35 percent of the total energy content. For those who participate in sport 20–25 percent is recommended to allow for increased carbohydrate levels.

Salt

The use of salt and salty food should also be moderated. Many New Zealanders continue to add salt to foods on the plate or consume a significant amount of salty foods. If using salt, select iodised salt and taste food before adding.

Include foods from all the four major food groups in the baseline eating programme, but take care with the proportion of fat, sweets and alcohol in your diet. Concentrate on obtaining the majority of your energy intake in the baseline eating pattern from the bread and cereals and the fruit and vegetables groups. Choose wholegrain and fresh alternatives where possible.

The use of meat and meat products should be kept to around three times a week and you should include more vegetarian meals in your diet. For example, try quiche with wholemeal pastry, rice dishes, pasta meals, stuffed baked potatoes, baked beans and other dried legumes.

Reduce the fat content of meals by removing all visible fat before cooking and using a minimal amount of butter on bread and toast. Scrape it on and scrape it off again.

Remember everyone is an individual. Work out a programme which best suits your needs or seek professional assistance. Try to eat regular meals. When meals are missed, coordinating your training schedule with a balanced eating pattern is difficult to achieve. Smaller, more frequent meals may be more suitable for some people.

By eating a wide variety of foods at regular times and maintaining a suitable body weight and composition, sports performance can only be enhanced.

Digestion processes

Once food leaves the plate it begins a journey through several of the body systems and is processed. After the food leaves the mouth once chewing has broken it into moist, easily swallowed pieces it is continually broken down into smaller and smaller units. For example, an apple which consists mainly of starch (a complex carbohydrate) breaks down until the chemical structures of glucose and fructose are reached. The starch in the apple is absorbed into the blood in the form of these two simple sugars. The digestive system cannot break them down any further. Any food which is not digested is passed out of the body (dietary fibre). The liver and muscles then convert the glucose (from the blood) into energy. Ultimately, the nutritional components of food end up performing some function that enables the person to use it for growth, repair, maintenance and energy. The process of digestion is illustrated below.

Digestion

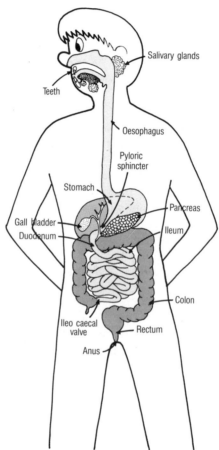

2
Body weight

For each person involved in sport there is an optimum weight range within which performance excels. This weight varies from person to person and according to age, sex, sport and so on. It also varies as individuals grow and develop their sports. An athlete or sportsperson who is overweight places general health at risk by increasing the potential to develop heart disease, diabetes, high blood pressure, back pain and injury. This can also hinder stamina and performance. Exercise is an excellent way to reduce or maintain body weight or body fat levels. By combining exercise and careful control of the energy content of the food eaten a balance can be achieved.

Special considerations are required for sportspeople when deciding on a reasonable weight range because of the extra muscle carried by some individuals. Although there is no exact ideal weight for any one individual, the sportsperson can work out a suitable weight range which feels the most comfortable. A lightweight rower is required to compete in a specific weight class while maintaining strength. However, a gymnast is often required to minimise body weight while maximising strength and skill. A rugby player requires a higher proportion of lean tissue (muscle), weight and strength but the level varies depending on the position played; for example, a lock has different requirements from a winger. A bodybuilder concentrates on developing a higher proportion of muscle size while the weightlifter is more concerned with strength.

It is important to be able to determine a suitable weight relatively accurately. But more important is the maintenance of the desirable or ideal weight. Many people, including the competitive sportsperson, the casual athlete and the non-active, struggle to maintain weight at a suitable level. In fact, the loss of weight is a billion dollar industry in the US.

The term 'ideal' or 'desirable' is often referred to in weight tables and by professionals. This refers to the right balance or combination of muscle, bone and fat. It involves a series of measurements, not just a person's weight. Proportions of muscle, bone and fat should be in balance for the sportsperson to achieve strength plus sufficient size and energy to meet the specific demands of a particular sport without excess fat. To meet these demands, changes in body proportion of muscle and fat may be required. It is very important that competitive sport participants do not reduce the energy levels of their baseline or training eating programmes too drastically in order to produce weight reduction or weight maintenance, or this will reduce the energy available for exercise and will hinder training, reduce performance and induce early fatigue.

There are several methods used to measure or assess body weight. These include using weight-for-height tables, body mass index calculations, the pinch test, visual evaluation and measurements of body fat levels (for example, anthropometric tests and underwater weighing).

The body's weight is composed of many different constituents. These include muscle, nerves, bone, ligaments, tendons, skin, minerals, organs and fat. Some of these have the ability to change and others remain fixed. These constituents can be divided into two major parts: lean body weight (muscle, tissue and fat-free weight) and fat weight. Total body weight equals lean body weight plus fat weight.

There are marked sex differences in the body composition. In theory, the average man is taller, heavier, carries a larger and heavier skeleton, has a larger muscle mass and his total body fat is lower than the average woman's. Body fat represents 15–17 percent of a man's total body weight and 25–27 percent of a woman's. These frameworks are used to compare individuals in terms of body composition. They are not fixed values. There are differences between these reference figures for non-athletes and athletes. Athletes tend to be leaner and the percentage fat value varies according to the type of activity.

Body fat is divided into two groups. Essential fat is that stored in the marrow of bones, in the heart, lungs, liver, spleen, kidneys, intestines, muscles and nervous system. The fat found in these areas is essential for the normal functioning of the body. In females it is

■ *BODY FAT LEVELS IN DIFFERENT INDIVIDUALS*

Type of person		Fat level (%)
Woman:	average non-athletic	26
	athlete	12–20
	distance athlete	15–19
	bodybuilder	10
Man:	average non-athletic	15
	athlete	8–12
	distance athlete	6–18
	bodybuilder	4–6

■ ■ ■

there to provide some of the sex-related characteristic fat deposits, such as fullness in the breast, pelvic and thigh regions.

The other type of fat is storage fat. This is the fat that accumulates in the adipose tissue. Storage fat includes the fat that is laid down to protect the internal organs by acting as a buffer to possible injury, and the large deposits of subcutaneous (under the skin surface) fat. The total amount of this type of fat is four times higher in females than in males. This additional fat is important during pregnancy.

There appears to be a limit below which a sportsman's or sportswoman's body weight cannot be reduced without impairing health. For example, prior to competition bodybuilders severely restrict the intake of food, particularly carbohydrates, to reduce body fat levels to the extreme. It is important to remember that these very low levels should be maintained only for very short periods of time and are only achieved by the most dedicated. Low body fat levels have also been reported in marathon runners. This is a response to the high mileage and resulting energy expenditure in endurance training.

Assessing body composition

Not all body tissues contribute equally to the total weight of the body. The tissues which make up the lean body weight are more dense than the fat weight. For example, two sportswomen of the same height may be of the same weight, but looking at them it may be seen that one woman carries more fat weight.

Body composition measurements provide additional information for establishing weight loss, weight gain and exercise programmes and

21

a desired weight can be calculated. There are no formal guidelines for ideal percentages of body fat as this varies depending on the sport in which the athlete participates.

There are several methods available to assess the proportion of lean body weight. Some involve measuring the circumference of certain body parts such as the arm, thigh and calf with a measuring tape. Others measure the thickness of a pinch of skin and the surface fat in areas such as the arm, triceps, back and hips. Body density tests using underwater weighing techniques or electrical impulses are other methods.

A simple method you can carry out yourself is the mirror test. This is a purely subjective, unscientific method that involves removing the bulk of your clothes in front of a mirror and examining your reflection. Ask the following questions: Is your waist larger than your hips? Pinch the underside of your left arm and pull the skin and fat away from the muscle. More than 2 cm requires action. Repeat the pinch test with the waist. Do you approve of what you see? Although these tests are not reliable they do allow you to make an initial evaluation.

Height/weight charts

Height/weight charts apply to the general population but provide a poor guide for the highly trained or elite sportsperson. This is a particularly important consideration for bodybuilders, power lifters, rugby players and other sportspeople who carry a higher proportion of lean muscle. These charts can make the sportsperson appear overweight or even obese.

Some individuals who fall at the upper end of the range may find it necessary to reduce weight or body fat percentage. These ranges are generous and anyone falling outside them will need to make some changes.

Weight measurements include all the body weight and do not provide any indication of the quality of weight carried by an individual. As muscle weighs more than fat and people who engage in regular exercise or activity have more lean body weight (muscle), these people may seem overweight when in fact they are a healthy weight.

Body mass index (BMI)

BMI indicates a healthy weight range using body height (in metres), squared, and weight (in kilograms). This measurement is often used in hospitals and can be effectively adapted for people active in sport. These measurements require some interpretation. Use BMI in conjunction with other measurements for sports participants.

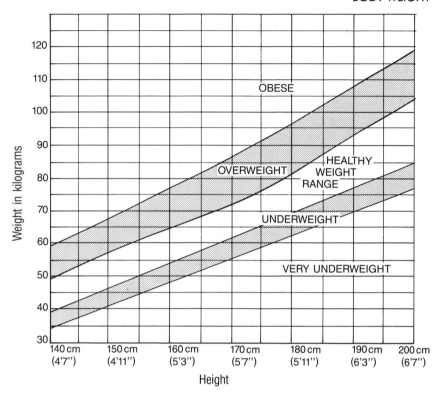

Weight for height chart for men and women

(Reproduced with the permission of the Australian Nutrition Foundation.)

■ WEIGHT RANGES FOR ADULTS AGED 20-60 YEARS

Height m	Weight kg	
	Women	Men
1.50	42–52	45–53
1.55	45–55	48–58
1.60	48–58	50–62
1.65	52–62	53–65
1.70	54–67	56–69
1.75	58–70	59–73
1.80	62–75	63–78
1.85	66–80	70–82

(Nutrition Advisory Committee, *Recommendations for Selected Nutrient Intakes for New Zealanders, 1983.*)

■ ■ ■

23

$$BMI = \frac{weight\ (kg)}{height\ (m)^2}$$

Under 18   severely underweight
18–20   underweight
20–25   healthy weight range
25–30   overweight
Over 30   severely overweight
(Note: values are for the non-athlete)

■ EXAMPLES

A 55 kg (8½ st) female middle distance runner is concerned that she is carrying excess fat. On visual interpretation she appears within her weight range. She is 1.57 m tall (5 ft 2 in).

$$\frac{55}{(1.57 \times 1.57)} = \frac{55}{2.46}$$

$$= 22.3\ (healthy\ weight)$$

If this woman were a gymnast, ballet dancer, jockey, or lightweight rower it might be necessary to consider some form of mild reduction in weight.

Consider a 1.92 m (6 ft 2 in) front row rugby player who weighs 101.5 kg (16 st).

BMI

$$\frac{101.5}{(1.92 \times 1.92)} = \frac{101.5}{3.68}$$

$$= 27.5$$

Again this method does not indicate the quality of weight and values appear inappropriate for some sports. Technically this front row forward is overweight but visual assessment and body fat percentages indicate a higher proportion of muscle. These values do not apply to children or adolescents.

Body circumference

Body fat can be calculated by using a tape measure to record the circumference of certain body sites. The body sites measured include the upper arm, waist and forearm. Age and sex are taken into consideration.

Although these measurements are easy to obtain they may not be valid for athletic men or women, or for very thin or obese individuals.

The measurement of body composition can provide useful information to determine a desirable weight. This is a more individual approach than referring to tables of ideal weights. Skinfold measurements used in conjunction with height/weight data can provide more information.

Hydrostatic (underwater) weighing

Much controversy exists over the accuracy of the methods used to measure body composition. This method is considered to be one of the more precise laboratory techniques. The athlete is weighed twice, once in the air and the second time submerged in water. Athletes with a higher percentage of fat will weigh less underwater. These two weights allow the calculation of a percentage body fat. It is a time-consuming and generally uncomfortable procedure. The availability of this form of assessment is limited to specialised centres and can be expensive because of equipment and technical costs. It is important to remember that although this method is reasonably accurate, underwater weighing can be in error by plus or minus 2–3 percent body fat. In addition, people have different levels of bone density, which alters the equations used to determine percentage body fat. However, despite the limitations of this method it is used to compare with other body composition measurement methods and provides a reasonable indicator of percentage fat.

Skinfold measurements

These pinch tests provide an easy measurement to estimate the percentage of body fat. The skinfold thickness (pinching a fold of

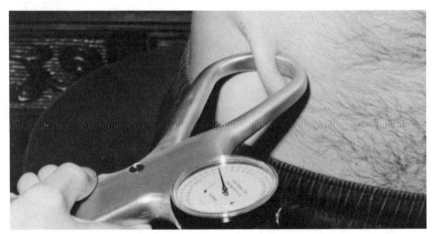

Performing skinfold measurements on athletes requires skill and accuracy as some have low body fat levels due to training and the specific demands of their sport.

skin) is measured at various points around the body using callipers. Calculations are made considering both age and sex. In some cases, the sport of a specific athlete requires consideration regarding the location of deposits of fat. Care and accuracy in measurement are essential for valid readings. Generally, five body sites are assessed although there is some support for a seven-site assessment. Changes in skinfold measurements (or percentages of body fat) can be used to assess weight reduction programmes. However, accurate measurements in obese people are more difficult to obtain. The method requires minimal equipment, a high degree of skill and consistent measurement taking. It is the most convenient and least stressful of all the methods.

Bio-electrical impedance analysis (BIA)

Another technique, which uses electrical currents to estimate the percentage of body fat, is BIA. The readings are based on the resistance to the electrical current. The higher the proportion of lean tissue the less electrical resistance. This method, not available in New Zealand, remains controversial and expensive. Measurements are affected by changes in body water; for example, the use of diuretics, consumption of alcohol, oedema or fluid retention, dehydration or sweating from exercise will all influence results.

The most practical and inexpensive method to determine weight status and body composition is the skinfold measurement. This provides estimates of body fat percentages and when used with the BMI and visual appraisal realistic assessments can be made.

3
Carbohydrates

Carbohydrates are the most efficient and effective source of fuel for sportspeople. They are made from the chemicals carbon, hydrogen and oxygen and supply ready-made energy for exercise. Carbohydrates are taken into the body and 'burned' with oxygen to release energy; the process is similar to burning petrol in a car. Before the muscle cells can use carbohydrates they must be broken down into simpler, smaller units such as glucose.

Glucose is one of the simplest forms of carbohydrate and is transferred around the body in the blood. It is used by the muscle for energy, stored as glycogen in the liver and used by the brain and other tissues of the body. Glycogen is stored as fuel in the body just as starch is stored in plants. Glycogen is converted back into glucose to be used for energy when required.

Carbohydrates are classified as either simple or complex. Simple sugars are generally easily digested and absorbed and will rapidly raise blood sugar levels compared to complex sugars — an important consideration for performance. The sugars in fruit, jam and honey, table sugar (raw, white, brown, icing and castor), and milk are all converted to simple sugars (glucose, fructose and galactose). Complex carbohydrate foods include cereals (wheat, corn, oats), rice, bread, pasta, fruit and vegetables. These foods are also high in other nutrients, especially fibre, vitamins and minerals. Maintaining an adequate energy (kilojoule) intake is essential for maximum performance.

Complex carbohydrates are often referred to as starches and are usually of plant origin. The eating patterns for anyone who regularly participates in sports should involve mainly carbohydrates of the complex form. Wholegrain and wholemeal varieties are preferred for general health, although as dietary fibre is not absorbed it is not considered a source of energy for sportspeople. Because of their slower absorption rates from the small intestines into the bloodstream during digestion, complex carbohydrates do not generally produce a rapid rise in blood sugars.

Carbohydrate foods are inexpensive, readily available and easily metabolised, which makes them the ideal fuel for the body. Carbohydrates also have several unique properties that make them the number one energy source. They are the only foods that can be broken down and used by the body (metabolised) without oxygen (anaerobically).

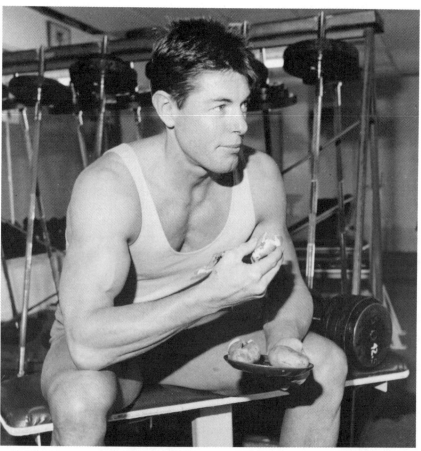

As a bodybuilder, Leo Quintus recognises the importance of maintaining carbohydrate intakes during bouts of intense training.

The greatest turnover of carbohydrate for energy occurs during the first few minutes of moderate to heavy activity and the fuel for this is provided by blood glucose. Then the glycogen stored in the liver and muscle takes over. As glycogen is used for activity, an increase in fat oxidation (burning) or gluconeogenesis (making glucose from storage) occurs in the liver. Liver glycogen regulates the level of blood glucose while the stores of muscle glycogen provide the muscle with energy during the exercise.

Around 8.4 megajoules (MJ) of energy is stored as carbohydrate in the body and over 58.8 MJ of energy is stored as fat. Therefore, eating carbohydrate foods will not result in gaining weight if exercise is balanced. Most of the extra kilojoules come from the fat and sugar (butter and jam) eaten with carbohydrate foods. Below are examples of the amount of carbohydrate found in some common foods.

■ CARBOHYDRATE CONTENT OF SOME COMMON FOODS

Food	Carbohydrate %	Food	Carbohydrate %
Sugar	100	Fruit yoghurt	11
Rice	87	Feijoas	11
White flour	80	Grapefruit	10
Sweet syrups	79	Beetroot	6
Dates	76	Tamarillos	6
Raisins	75	Milk	5
Currants	73	Kamokamo	4
Wholegrain flour	73	Cottage cheese	3
White bread	55	Spinach	3
Biscuits	53	Watercress	0
Wholegrain bread	47	Puha	0
Pancakes	36	Meat	0
Baked beans	22	Fish	0
Hamburger	16	Cheese	0
Apples	12	Eggs	0

Carbohydrates and exercise

Glucose is the primary carbohydrate used for energy by exercising muscles. Factors that influence the use of carbohydrates for exercise are: duration and intensity of exercise, initial glycogen levels, muscles used, diet and hormone levels. With moderate to heavy exercise glycogen levels are rapidly metabolised for energy in the first few minutes; this tends to slow down to a steady rate until low levels are reached. At low levels of exercise muscle glycogen is used slowly and glycogen stores are not necessarily depleted to exhaustion.

There are two distinct types of muscle fibres: the fast-twitch and the slow-twitch. Fast-twitch fibres are used for high speed and short periods of time. Sprinting uses predominantly these muscle fibres. The fuel source is carbohydrates and lactic acid is produced. These fibres contract rapidly and fatigue easily. As the lactic acid gradually builds up it inhibits muscle contraction.

Slow-twitch fibres are longer, contract slower and keep going for longer periods of time. These fibres are less powerful, as they work at a lower level of effort. Carbohydrates and fats are required for fuel. These are the fibres used for endurance activities. During high intensity exercise fast-twitch muscle fibres use more glycogen than slow-twitch fibres. Trained athletes use glycogen at a slower rate than the untrained when performing the same level of moderate intensity exercise. This may be the result of an increased ability to use fat as a fuel source and the influence of hormone levels.

There are three methods the body can use to maintain blood glucose levels when no carbohydrate foods have been eaten and there is no absorption of glucose from the digestive system. Fat is used as the preferred source of energy by muscle and other tissues. Glycogen which has been stored in the liver is released and converted to glucose and the liver also has the ability to produce glucose from protein. This occurs in cases of fasting or starvation, but it does have a detrimental effect on fuel sources and body tissues. However, no harm results from a short-term fast, such as overnight.

When comparing the effect of a high fat diet, a mixed diet and a high carbohydrate diet researchers discovered that athletes consuming a high carbohydrate diet were able to exercise longer — twice as long as the mixed diet exercisers and three times longer than those eating a high fat diet. The initial levels of glycogen at the onset of exercise are important in determining the length of time moderate to heavy exercise can be sustained.

The practice by some sports participants of ingesting concentrated glucose solutions (greater than 2.5 percent) prior to competition does not appear to enhance performance. In fact, if these solutions are taken 45 minutes before exercise they can actually result in poor performance and can lower blood sugar levels after about 30 minutes of exercise. (See chapter 12.) Eating or drinking concentrated glucose solutions or foods (sugar solutions, chocolate-coated candy bars) immediately before exercise should be avoided.

Foods that increase carbohydrate intake

New Zealanders are encouraged to reduce intakes of sugars and increase other sources of carbohydrate. To achieve this nutritional goal eat some form of carbohydrate food at each meal. This includes bread, rice, cereals, pasta, potato, macaroni, fruit and vegetables. Other suggestions include dried fruit and nuts, sandwiches and plain crackers. Try not to add sugar to foods, and eat regular meals. Eating some form of carbohydrate food two to three hours (this time frame is subject to individual variation) before training and exercise will enhance energy levels by stabilising blood glucose levels and improve performance. Although it is desirable to increase the intake of wholegrain bread, a corresponding increase in butter, jam and honey is not acceptable.

The following foods are high in carbohydrate with a moderate to low fat content.

Breads, rolls, buns: all wholemeal varieties.

Rice: used as a savoury item or as rice pudding made with trim milk and fruit.

Pasta: spaghetti and all forms of noodles, but take care with the sauces.

Legumes: including bean salads and baked beans.

Plain biscuits, crackers and a few unroasted nuts.

All fruits: fresh or dried without added sugar, including fruit juices.

All vegetables: especially potatoes (not roasted, fried or as chips), pumpkin, kumara, parsnip, peas, sweetcorn, yams, beetroot, broad beans, carrots and mixed vegetables.

Most cereals: rice bubbles, cornflakes, porridge, muesli (watch for added oil, sugar or honey), Weetbix, Puffed Wheat, All Bran and bran flakes. As muesli bars can be high in sugar or honey, check the food label.

Complex carbohydrates are the most valuable source of energy for sports participants and increase glycogen stores more efficiently than simple carbohydrates. Fats and proteins play only a minor role in energy release and carbohydrates are the preferred fuel for exercise.

4
Sugar

Sugar is sugar — whether it is white, brown, raw, or in a syrup, cube or powder. The body does not distinguish between the various sources of sugar. There are many pros and cons for including sugar in the diet, as well as some unresolved and controversial ideas concerning the role of sugar in health. For the sportsperson, sugar is often seen as a readily available source and supplier of energy and several foods are marketed on this concept, in particular some forms of chocolate-coated candy bars. However, there are a number of health problems caused by the consumption of excess sugar; these include dental caries or tooth decay, and here it is more important how often the sugar is eaten than the amount. Excess weight is another problem and this is a consequence of too much sugar or foods containing sugar.

One of the recommendations in *Nutritional Guidelines for New Zealanders* (see Bibliography) is to reduce sugar intake. The annual average sugar intake is high. There has been little change in the total amount of sugar consumed by New Zealanders since 1900. Over one year the average New Zealander can expect to eat around 48 kg of sugar. This works out to be 900 g or almost 1 kg per week — an incredible half a cup per day. These figures include not only the fine white powder sprinkled on cereals and put into beverages but also sugar used in manufactured goods such as baked products (cakes, pastries and biscuits), jams, soft drinks and alcohol. Over 60 percent of all sugar produced ends up in a manufactured product. Manufacturers aware of the concern over excessive sugar are producing a number of products labelled 'no added sugar'. This suggests to the consumer that they may be lower in kilojoules. The sugar present may be in the form of corn syrup, treacle, glucose or added fruit juice, but there may be no significant difference in kilojoule levels of these foods.

There have been some changes in the types of sugar eaten. Although white sugar still dominates it has decreased about 15 percent. This change has been compensated for by an increase in brown and raw sugar. In Australia, the average intake of sugar is about 50 kg per person per year while Americans consume 34 kg per person per year. In addition to their sugar intake Americans consume another 21 kg as corn syrup. This brings their total to 55 kg. We must not forget the honey used or the golden syrup and treacle spread on crumpets and added to cooking and drinks. This all adds to our total sugar consumption.

Sugar is a low nutrient density food. This means it does not provide any other nutrients to the body apart from energy (or kilojoules). Sugar is also low in fibre, which makes it an easy food to overeat. There are many advertisements portraying high sugar foods as good sources of energy. The Homestyle survey suggested an increase of 25 percent in chocolate consumption from 1980 to 1984. In 1983 around 20 million candy bars were eaten in New Zealand. This is an average of 25 per person, which means that, on average, each New Zealander devours approximately 8 kg of lollies each year.

The chemical name for table sugar is sucrose. This is a mixture of glucose and fructose chemically joined together. Sucrose is broken down by the digestive system into glucose and fructose before it can be absorbed into the bloodstream. The blood then transports the glucose to areas of the body where it is needed (such as the muscle) and stores the leftover as fat.

Excessive amounts of sugar, especially glucose, consumed before a competition or game can have a detrimental effect on performance. When high intakes of sugar (sucrose) are digested and enter the bloodstream a hormone called insulin is released. If this occurs during exercise the blood sugar of the sportsperson is drastically lowered owing to the combined effect of exercise and insulin. This causes early fatigue, inhibiting performance. A moderate intake of starch-based or complex carbohydrate foods that have a lesser effect on blood sugars is recommended. The energy value of sugar is 84 kJ or 20 Cal per teaspoon. If a person were to drink a cup of tea or coffee with one teaspoon of sugar, six times a day, in one year they would have helped themselves to 2 190 teaspoons or 11 kg of sugar. This would add up to 504 kJ per day, 3 528 kJ per week, or 183 500 kJ per year. This will add 12½ lb or 5½ kg to the waistline in one year, unles you have used up these kilojoules in exercise. It's all a matter of balance.

It is not necessary to ban sugar altogether from the diet but it is important to moderate the intake. Use the sweetness found naturally in foods and do not add sugar to fruit drinks and stewed fruits. Limit the eating of sweets and foods high in sugar to special occasions and with meals rather than as snacks or between meals.

White sugar, brown sugar, raw sugar, honey, golden syrup, treacle and maple syrup all have very similar nutritional compositions weight for weight. Golden syrup, corn syrup, molasses, maple syrup and honey are all liquid sugars. They contain more water than is found in the dry forms. Be careful of the amount of liquid sugars used. As a liquid they are easier to spread and it is easy to add more in cooking, which increases the energy content of the food.

Soft drinks, cakes and biscuits all contain large amounts of hidden sugar. A can of fizzy drink may contain up to 9 teaspoons of sugar. Read the labels on the back of packets and canned foods for added sugar, remembering that sugar can be disguised as honey, malt, sucrose, glucose, lactose (milk sugar), corn syrup, or any combination of the above. White sugar is one of the purest sugars and is 99.9 percent sucrose. Honey contains 19 percent water, 2 percent sucrose, 34 percent glucose and 40 percent fructose. Use less jam, marmalade and honey on bread, toast and sandwiches.

It is important to remember also that if weight gain is desired this is no licence to eat more sugar and sugar-containing foods.

How to reduce sugar intake

The following suggestions are offered as a guideline to reduce the intake of sugar:

- Where possible use the fresh alternative, for example, fresh fruit to replace fruit juice. It is very easy to drink a litre of fruit juice in a day but hard work to eat 10 to 12 apples. One cup of undiluted fruit juice equals three slices of bread in energy value. Dilute fruit juice at least 50/50 with water.

- Limit the number of glasses of sweet cordials and soda drink each day.

- Drink more water. Add slices of lemon and fresh mint to improve the taste of the water.

- Use herbs and spices to flavour foods instead of adding sugar. Vanilla essence can also be used.

■ *AVERAGE PERCENTAGE OF SUGAR CONTENT IN SELECTED FOODS*

Type of food	%	Type of food	%
Peppermints	99	Milk chocolate	57
Wine gums	89	Muesli bar	37
Jam	70	Ice cream	22
Dark chocolate	60		

■ ■ ■

■ *SUGAR CONTENT AND ENERGY VALUE OF SOME COMMON FOODS*

Quantity	Food	Sugar g	Kilojoules
1 cup	chocolate milkshake	40	1270
1 glass	white wine	10	928
1 x 100 g	muesli bar	18–20	627–920
1 cup	fruit juice	28–30	502
1 glass	cola soft drink	26	439
1 cup	whole milk	12	355
1 cup	fruit juice (no added sugar)	18–20	301
1 cup	tea with 1 teaspoon sugar	5	84

■ ■ ■

- Use artificial sweeteners only as a last resort or to sweeten food occasionally. These are not recommended for children.

- A little sugar once in a while does no harm but save sugar and high sugar foods for treats rather than consuming them on a regular basis.

- Use less jam, marmalade, honey and lemon spreads on breakfast toast and sandwiches. These are almost pure sugar.

- Read the labels on cereal packets. Look for added sugar listed as sucrose, honey, malt, lactose, glucose. This includes foods such as muesli and muesli bars.

- Maintain nutritional intake through eating a wide variety of foods.

- Reduce the amount of sugar added to foods in baking and at the table.

- Reduce the amount of sugar added to drinks. Drink tea and coffee without sugar. Reducing the amount of coffee added reduces the bitter taste. Try tea made a little weaker and brewed for a shorter time.

Sugar and exercise

Not all carbohydrates are equivalent in enhancing performance. Although the major portion of the pre-game meal should be composed of carbohydrate, the ingestion of some forms (glucose) taken in excessive amounts is not recommended.

The ingestion of glucose causes a dramatic increase in blood insulin levels before exercise commences. The function of insulin is to reduce blood glucose levels to normal. However, as exercise uses blood glucose levels for fuel the combination of increased insulin and exercise leads to progressively lower blood glucose levels or hypoglycaemia. Feelings of fatigue occur and greater dependence must be placed on muscle glycogen levels as fuel for the exercise or sports performance. Muscle glycogen levels are, therefore, depleted sooner during endurance activities, resulting in earlier muscular fatigue and diminished performance.

For any activity lasting under two hours, water is the preferred liquid. Any liquid containing sugar or glucose must be diluted to 2.5 g per 100 ml and consumed up to one hour before performance. Some vegetable juices may be a suitable alternative, but care must be taken with the sodium content. Fruit juices should be diluted. For events lasting longer than two hours, such as the Ironman or Coast-to-coast, special considerations apply. (These are specifically addressed on page 165.)

Artificial sweeteners

If you want to lose a kilogram or a few pounds and are counting your kilojoules or calories you may decide to replace sugar with an artificial sweetener. These are compounds which have a sweet taste but little or no nutritive value or energy.

There are several varieties on the market today. Saccharine is approximately 300 times sweeter than sugar, aspartame 200 times sweeter and cyclamate 30 times sweeter. Saccharine and cyclamate have been used to replace sugar for a number of years and are added to a wide range of foods including drinks, desserts, salad dressings and ice cream. Saccharine has been around for about 80 years without any apparent harmful effects to humans.

In the 1970s both saccharine and cyclamate were banned in America. Very high doses had been fed to rats, a few of which developed bladder cancer. However, in these experiments 100 times the dose consumed by humans was fed to the rats. This would be equivalent to drinking 875 cans of artificially sweetened soft drink a day. The very small amounts commonly used in foods have not been shown to be harmful. In fact diabetics have been using them for years without any apparent side-effects.

The latest sweetener, Nutrasweet, or aspartame, is composed of proteins and no detrimental side-effects have been reported. The only limitation to using aspartame is that it contains the amino acid phenylalanine. A few people suffering from the rare disease phenylketonuria (PKU) are unable to metabolise this amino acid correctly. It is very important, especially for children suffering from PKU, that products containing aspartame are identified.

The use of articifial sweeteners has increased over the last few years as people act on recommendations to reduce sugar intake and maintain ideal body weight. But is this a help or does it just make us feel less guilty about eating sweet foods? The few calories less in a glass of artificially sweetened soda are often exceeded on chips, chocolate, desserts and cream.

There is no evidence that artificial sweeteners are useful in weight reduction and in the reduction of energy intake. An extensive study carried out in 1986 on the use of artificial sweeteners investigated the weight changes of middle-aged American women. Investigators reported that users of artificial sweeteners were more likely to gain weight. The use of sweeteners increased with weight and decreased with age. In the long term, the use of these sweeteners neither reduced nor prevented weight gain. The average difference in weight between users and non-users of artificial sweeteners was less than two pounds.

Even though it has never been proved that artificial sweeteners help dieters to reduce weight, let alone keep it off, sales of these items and the foods containing them continue to grow. The basic eating patterns have not changed. We stroll down supermarket aisles seeking out the lower kilojoule versions of favourite foods so we can continue to eat sweet and often high fat foods with less guilt. This way we can have twice as much without changing our eating habits. We are good at finding convenient substitutes that allow us to continue eating as we have always done, and manufacturers are very quick to provide these substitutes.

Before you replace sugar and high calorie foods with artificial low calorie alternatives, consider the following recommendations:

● Aim to make long-term changes to eating patterns.

● Use artificial sweeteners to help reduce the amount of sweetness you are accustomed to. Initially they can be used to replace the sugar added to beverages such as tea and coffee. Aim to reduce their use and adapt the taste buds to less sweet foods. Drink tea and coffee weaker and reduce bitterness by adding more water or milk.

- Drink more plain water instead of tea or coffee.

- Using artificial sweeteners will not discourage a sweet tooth. Learn to enjoy the natural sweetness of food without adding extra sugar or sweeteners. Try fresh fruit, dried fruit (not crystallised or candied), diluted fruit juices and yoghurt with unsweetened fruit.

- Using low calorie dressings will help reduce the calorie level of the meal or salad, but it is better to educate the taste buds to require less.

- Take smaller servings of favourite foods like ice cream and desserts. Eat these foods less often and enjoy them rather than continuing to eat the artificial reduced-calorie food regularly.

- Eat many different foods high in complex carbohydrate and low in fat, such as fresh fruits and vegetables. Regular exercise also plays a significant role in health and weight maintenance so continue activity through the off-season.

- Remember that artificial sweeteners do not contribute any energy or carbohydrate to a sports participant's food intake. They contain no fuel to burn.

5
Fat

In *Nutritional Guidelines for New Zealanders* it is recommended that we should reduce our intake of fat. However, as there are several different types of fat, we need to know which types to reduce and by how much. We also need to know the relevance of fat in the diet of the person actively engaged in exercise and sports activities.

Heart disease remains the principal cause of death for New Zealanders. Over 12 000 New Zealanders die each year from cardiovascular diseases. Despite the fact that the rate of death from heart disease has fallen by about one-third since the late 1960s, the level is still high, especially when compared to similar developed countries. Results of various research studies indicate that firm management of blood lipids (fats) can have a significant benefit to health. The proportion of saturated fat contained in the food we eat regularly is an area of serious concern and must be reduced.

Improvements can be made in several areas: reducing excess body fat, lowering blood cholesterol, reducing saturated fats and increasing participation in regular exercise. All assist in reducing the risk factors for heart disease and improve overall nutritional status.

Categories of food fats

Saturated fats are generally of animal origin, such as butter, lard, cream, dripping and the fat from meat. **Unsaturated fats** are the plant oils and include peanut, avocado, sunflower, olive and safflower oils and margarine. Unsaturated fats can be further divided into two more groups, **monounsaturated** and **polyunsaturated**. And just when it seems all sorted out two more fats appear on the scene — the **omega 3** and **omega 6** fats, which appear in some fish, particularly salmon, tuna and deep-sea fish.

■ FAT CONTENT OF COMMONLY USED OILS

Oil	Monounsaturated	Polyunsaturated	Saturated
Olive	***	*	*
Rapeseed	***	**	*
Corn	**	**	*
Soya bean	*	**	*
Sunflower	*	***	*
Safflower	*	***	*
Coconut	*	*	***
Palm kernel	*	*	***

* Low (less than 30%)
** Moderate (30–60%)
*** High (more than 60%)

■ ■ ■

Two vegetable fats, coconut and palm oil, which are high in saturated fat and low in unsaturated fats are used often in manufactured baked products. Check food labels for these foods listed in the first two ingredients.

The wide publicity about fat and the role of excessive intakes of saturated fats in some diseases (heart disease, stroke, non-insulin-dependent diabetes and some cancers) has produced a common belief that all fat is bad for health. However, two of the groups of fats, fish oils and monounsaturated oils, can actually improve health when included in moderate amounts as part of the total eating pattern.

Fats also provide a way for the body to obtain fat soluble vitamins (particularly vitamins A, D and E). These are essential for normal growth and the functioning of all tissues. Following an extreme low fat diet for long periods of time without paying attention to the quality of food eaten may result in a deficiency in some of these fat soluble vitamins. Also, the essential fatty acids (linoleic and linolenic acid) cannot be produced by the body but are supplied through the fat eaten in our diet. They are essential for growth and maintenance of a healthy skin. Therefore, some fat is necessary as part of a balanced and varied eating pattern.

Does avoiding fat keep you thin?

Fat contains the highest number of kilojoules or calories gram for gram when compared with protein, carbohydrates and even alcohol. One gram of fat provides 9 Cal, or 38 kJ. As a result it is very easy to overeat foods containing fat and become overweight. The body stores energy for later use as fat. Half a kilogram or 1 lb of excess body weight equals 14.7 megajoules (MJ) (3 500 Cal) of stored energy. Limiting the intake of foods with a high fat level and reducing added fat can help reduce body weight. Some researchers indicate that it is much easier to store body fat directly from fat eaten in the diet than it is to convert carbohydrates into body fat.

New Zealanders generally consume more fat than is necessary for good health. Some people actually prefer the flavour of higher fat foods. The addition of sugar (such as creamed butter and sugar or chocolate) makes the food more palatable. Eating patterns that are high in fat and cholesterol tend to be associated with higher fat levels in the blood, which may increase the risk of heart disease. This is important, particularly for those people with a high degree of risk factors (smoking, being overweight and a family history of heart disease). It has been estimated that over half the New Zealand population have a cholesterol level above the recommended ratio. For the general population, levels below 5.5 mmol/l (millimoles per litre) are recommended.

The key issue is the total amount of fat in the eating plan. Although most New Zealanders consume an average of 40 percent of their total kilojoules (or proportion of the energy value of the food eaten) as fat, the recommendations suggest that no more than 30 percent should consist of fat. For the sportsperson, increasing the carbohydrate portion of the diet to 60 percent leads to a decrease in fat intake down to 25 percent.

Fat makes up between 20 and 30 percent (usually 24–26 percent) of a female's body weight and between 10 and 15 percent of a male's. Females have more fat on their bodies than males. Fat is needed to protect the body's organs (kidney, liver, spleen) and provide a layer of insulation against cold or shock. The additional fat carried by women is thought to be provided for childbearing and hormone-related functions. Women should not reduce their body fat levels below 10–12 percent for long periods of time. A body fat of 15 percent is a suitable guideline for endurance athletes. A low body fat does not ensure an elite athlete.

When engaged in light to moderate (aerobic) exercise stored fat provides 50–60 percent of the energy used; as the activity continues this increases to 70 percent. This spares the glycogen reserves.

41

For example: half a kilogram or 1 lb body fat equals 14.7 MJ. A 68 kg (150 lb) athlete has 10–20 percent of fat stores which provides 265–529 MJ of energy. Even the leanest of endurance athletes carry enough fat storage to meet the needs of strenuous exercise.

Types of fat in the body

Triglycerides

There are three fat sources available to the body — stored triglycerides, blood triglycerides and free fatty acids. Triglycerides are composed of one glycerol unit linked with three fatty acids and make up about 90 percent of the fat in the diet. Triglycerides vary according to the different fatty acids they contain. Stored throughout the body as fatty tissue, triglycerides are available as a fuel source in the form of free fatty acids in the bloodstream. Excessive intakes of both protein and carbohydrate can be processed to form triglycerides.

Fatty acids

These are chemical structures of carbon, hydrogen and oxygen in varying proportions. If there are no double bonds present in the molecule the fatty acid is saturated. Monounsaturated fat has one double bond while polyunsaturated has many double bonds. The presence and position of the double bonds has important effects on the properties and functions of fatty acids. Two fatty acids (linoleic and linolenic) are referred to as essential fatty acids as the body is unable to produce them from other fatty acids. These fatty acids must be supplied by the diet. They are important for normal growth, the function of all body cells, and the production of certain hormone-like structures in the body. Fatty acids can be rebuilt into triglycerides and taken to the muscle or liver, or to storage in the adipose tissue. Fatty acids are the major source of fat burned during exercise.

Omega 3 and **omega 6** are fatty acids whose properties are still not fully understood. The numbers three and six describe the position of the first double bond in a fatty acid. Omega 3 and omega 6 are still the subject of research, but it appears that these fatty acids may have a protective role in heart disease by reducing the risk of blood clotting and the levels of blood cholesterol and triglycerides. Omega 3 fatty acids became the subject of much interest when researchers examining the traditional high fat Eskimo diet (from seal and whale blubber) did not see a high incidence of heart disease.

Yet when Eskimos moved to a more Western diet their heart disease rates increased.

However, the benefit of omega 3 remains debatable. There have been reports of side-effects from taking supplements. By increasing the consumption of fish to two or three times a week as part of the normal varied diet a balance can be achieved.

Cholesterol

Cholesterol is a waxy type of fat which is unique to animal cells. It is not essential in the diet as the liver can produce what the body needs. The function of cholesterol is to make bile acids (important for the absorption of fats), cell membranes (including brain and nerve tissue), body hormones (particularly the sex hormones) and vitamin D. Most cholesterol in the body is produced from saturated fats rather than the cholesterol already present in food. Excessive intakes of saturated fats and food high in cholesterol increase the risk of developing high levels in the bloods which may result in the development of atherosclerosis (a condition where fatty deposits cause the narrowing and possible clotting of blood vessels). A blood test is used to measure blood cholesterol. A total cholesterol of 5.5 mmol/l has been set as the maximum, but this varies with age. The blood cholesterol for many New Zealanders is above the World Health Organisation recommendations (5.17 mmol/l).

There is growing evidence to suggest that regular physical exercise lowers cholesterol levels. Increases in blood levels of the cholesterol scavenger (high density lipoprotein or HDL), which removes cholesterol from the blood, have also been reported in groups of athletes. Exercise is encouraged as part of most coronary heart disease rehabilitation programmes.

The form of cholesterol which causes most concern is carried in the blood by the low density lipoprotein (LDL). It is the ratios between the HDL and LDL and the HDL and blood cholesterol levels which are important.

Fats and exercise

Your body stores energy as fat for later use. Fat is essential in the overall eating plan. Fats are also the most concentrated source of food energy. Weight for weight they provide more than twice the energy supplied by carbohydrates and protein.

Three factors that influence the use of fats during exercise are length of exercise, fitness and diet. In addition to the length of activity the intensity of exercise influences the use of fat for fuel. The degree of the sports participant's fitness and training influences the use of fat for fuel. Training increases the capacity of the body to burn fat during activity and enables free fatty acids to be mobilised and taken to the muscle during exercise. Free fatty acids are fat broken down to allow it to be utilised as a fuel source. Exercise performed at a high intensity for a short time will not utilise fat as a source of fuel. In the first few minutes of low to moderate intensity exercise glucose will be the primary fuel. There is a time lag between the onset of activity and switching from carbohydrate to fat for fuel.

Composition of the food eaten preceding exercise also influences the fuel source used for energy. If a high fat diet is consumed more energy will be used from fat while a high carbohydrate intake reduces the portion of fat used and increases the supply of carbohydrates for energy. Therefore, the presence of fat plays an important role in sparing (saving) carbohydrate, which is in limited supply as a source of fuel. In endurance exercise the body adapts and has the ability to use fats for energy and fuel, allowing the sportsperson or athlete to perform longer without exhaustion. However, this cannot be interpreted to mean that a high fat diet increases endurance. Carbohydrate from glycogen stores is still the preferred fuel.

Only stored triglycerides in fat storage and muscle are energy sources during exercise. The supply of fuel from blood trigylcerides is very small, but fat between muscles (intramuscular lipid stores) has been shown to decrease by 30–50 percent during 30–100 km races. Consuming a high fat diet causes a larger amount of fat to be used as fuel for exercise. Fatty acids from triglycerides storage are taken via the blood to the exercising muscle. Therefore, the concentration of free fatty acids will determine the amount available for the body to burn as fuel. During training, body fat levels are often reduced because fat stores are burned for energy. The size of the cells in the adipose tissue decreases without changing the actual number of cells. Fat cells do not change into muscle cells.

There are some problems with the use of high fat diets as these limit the amount of carbohydrate stored and this will eventually limit endurance. A high fat intake can reduce performance in sport. This is important as, although fats are a major source of fuel (energy) for endurance events, a fatty meal is slow to digest and leave the stomach. This can take up to four hours and an uncomfortable feeling of fullness may arise during activity.

Muscles cannot use fat as a primary source of fuel during exercise. There is a time lag in the first few minutes of exercise when the fatty acids are taken from storage and delivered to the muscles. During this time carbohydrates are used for fuel. It takes between 30 and

60 minutes before the fatty acids have increased to a sufficient level in the blood.

Training increases the capacity of the muscle to use fat. Some highly trained marathon runners exercising at 70 percent capacity for one hour have 75 percent of their fuel supplied from fat. But performance on high fat/low carbohydrate diets, when compared with high carbohydrate diets, is significantly impaired. Sportspeople and endurance athletes should avoid changing to a high fat diet low in carbohydrate during the depletion phase of carbohydrate loading before competition.

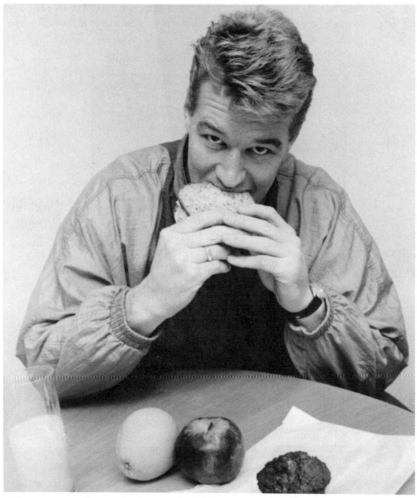

John Kirwan selects a high carbohydrate, low fat lunch to provide fuel for a training session.

Fats and health

Studies on several populations have shown a relationship between the amount of cholesterol consumed and deaths from heart disease. Blood cholesterol increases with raised levels of saturated fat. Increased fat levels in the diet raise total energy levels leading to overweight and obesity. This leads to inactivity and an increased incidence of high blood pressure and diabetes in susceptible individuals.

Regular aerobic exercise promotes the use of fat for fuel and decreases cholesterol and triglyceride levels in the blood. Well-trained athletes appear to have higher HDL levels in their blood; increased HDL levels are considered to reduce the risk of coronary heart disease.

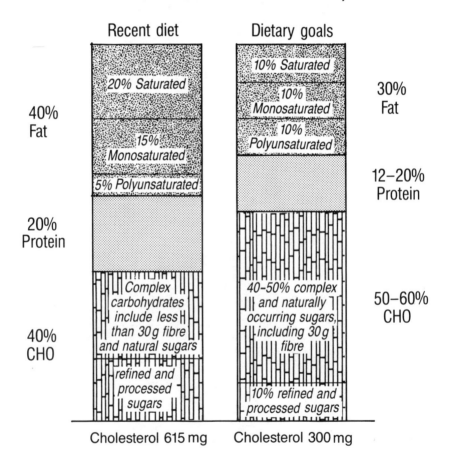

Dietary goals for New Zealanders.

It is recommended that you reduce your fat intake to 30 percent of total energy. The ideal combination is to lower saturated fat to 10 percent, increase polyunsaturated intake to 10 percent and use the monounsaturated fats to make up the remaining 10 percent. Increasing the fat content of the sportsperson's diet has no significant advantage and may impair performance.

■ *EXAMPLE OF THE FAT CONTENT OF SOME FOODS*

Food	Amount	Fat content g
Chicken roasted with skin	200 g	20
Chicken without skin	200 g	8
Fish in batter	100 g	18
Fish baked	100 g	1
Chop (1) with fat	180 g	44
Meat (fat trimmed)	¾ cup	11–12
Meat pie	1	24
Hamburger	1	14
Potato chips (hot)	½ cup	25
Potato chips (crisps)	50 g	18
Whole milk	1 cup	11
Trim milk	1 cup	1.2
Butter/margarine	1 tsp	4
Mashed potato with butter	½ cup	6
Avocado	2 tbsp	7
Cream	2 tbsp	12
Cheddar cheese (2 slices)	40 g	14
Cottage cheese	¼ cup	2
Fruit-flavoured yoghurt	½ cup	2
Apple/pear	1	*
Salad	1 cup	*
Fruit juice	1 cup	*
Cabbage, carrots, cauliflower	1 cup	*

* Indicates minimal or no fat present.

■ ■ ■

How to reduce fat intake

The following guidelines will help you to significantly reduce your fat intake.

● Use the low fat variety of a food. For example, use trim or skim milk, cottage cheese, quark, cheeses made with part skim milk, low fat yoghurts and oil-free dressing.

- Reduce the amount of butter, margarine, oil and cream added in cooking or used daily on muffins, bread or crackers.

- Grill, steam, boil, microwave and bake instead of frying and roasting.

- Trim the fat off all meat (including the skin on chicken) before cooking. Use lean meat such as trim pork, lean lamb and fish.

- In winter, when cooking a roast meal use water instead of fat or oil and roast one vegetable only. Try the vegetables in their jackets or wrapped in foil. Take care with gravy and white or cheese sauces.

- Replace some meat meals with legumes, such as dried beans and peas.

- Add more herbs, spices and other flavourings (for example, dried fruit) to meals instead of extra butter, gravy or cream.

- Take care with foods which have a high fat content. Have them only occasionally, as part of the meal plan, for a special treat. These foods include potato chips and crisps, roasted nuts, pastry, battered and fried fish, takeaways, rich cakes, buns, pastries and biscuits.

■ LOW FAT MENU

Breakfast	1 cup orange juice 4 Weetbix 1 cup trim milk 1 cup fresh fruit salad
Lunch	2 slices wholegrain bread 1 cup baked beans 1 cup salad vegetables 2 tsp margarine 2 tsp oil-free dressing 1 banana
Dinner	120 g baked fish 3 tbsp sweet-and-sour lemon sauce 1 baked potato 1 serving broccoli 1 serving carrots

1 cup fruit
1 cup low fat yoghurt

Snacks

2 fresh fruit
6 crackers with tomato
1 cup trim milk

Energy intake:	10.3 MJ	2 450 Cal
Carbohydrate:	71%	431 g
Protein:	17%	107 g
Fat:	12%	33 g

■ ■ ■

6
Protein

Although many people actively engaged in sport have heard the message to reduce their fat consumption, this message has been interpreted by some as a call to drastically limit their intake of red meat. As a result, many sportspeople have attempted to incorporate more vegetarian meals into their eating patterns. Reducing fat content is not a simple matter of cutting out all meats and replacing these with vegetables. The body has a specific requirement for essential amino acids which make up the various proteins in the body. In addition, meat, especially red meat, provides a number of minerals, the principle ones being iron, zinc and some calcium. By choosing the lower fat varieties of foods, especially meat and dairy products, intakes of protein can be maintained without increasing fat intake.

If you do choose to maintain a vegetarian diet ensure that the foods you select provide all the essential amino acids by combining legumes and grains effectively. (See chapter 17.)

There are many misunderstandings concerning the protein needs of sportspeople. Coaches, athletes and support personnel still believe that sportspeople require large quantities of protein for muscle growth and development. However, unlike carbohydrate and fat, protein has only a minor role as a source of energy during training and sports performance.

The principal function of protein is to build, maintain and repair body tissue, and to produce enzymes and some hormones. Protein makes up 20 percent of an individual's body weight and the majority of this is found in the muscle. As a person grows new cells are developed; throughout life these cells wear out and must be replaced.

This is the function of protein, the main body-building nutrient. Protein, with the assistance of vitamins, minerals, carbohydrate and fats, allows growth to take place.

Protein is made up of sub-units called amino acids. There are around 20 different amino acids and these combine in different ways to make different types of protein. Eight of these amino acids are essential for health in adults while 10 are essential for growth in children.

■ *THE ESSENTIAL AMINO ACIDS*

> Isoleucine
> Leucine
> Lysine
> Methionine
> Phenylalanine
> Threonine
> Tryptophan
> Valine
> Arginine — essential for children
> Histidine — essential for children

■ ■ ■

The protein molecule is made up of carbon, hydrogen and oxygen (like carbohydrate and fats), but it also contains nitrogen. Many of the body proteins also contain other elements such as sulphur, phosphorus and iron. Some of the proteins in the body include myosin (found in muscle), insulin (a hormone) and blood cells. Proteins which are found in foods are included in the following table:

■ *PROTEINS FOUND IN FOODS*

Collagen	meat and fish
Myosin	meat and fish
Elastin	meat
Caseln	milk and cheese
Lactalbumin	milk
Ovalbumin	egg white
Gluten	wheat

■ ■ ■

Most foods contain some protein. Bread, for example, is 10 percent protein, 2 g of protein per slice. Whole eggs are considered to contain the best quality of mixed amino acids, which explains why eggs are used as the standard to compare other sources of amino acids.

Protein needs for different individuals

Protein intake is calculated on a sportsperson's body weight with modifications for age and phase of growth. Requirements are increased further by pregnancy and breastfeeding. By estimating your protein requirement based on your body weight you can provide for a greater protein intake and increase muscle mass.

The following table gives the current recommended daily protein intake:

■ RECOMMENDED ADEQUATE DAILY INTAKE OF PROTEIN FOR NEW ZEALANDERS

Infants under 1 year	2 g/kg
Children	35–50 g
Young women (9–17 years)	51–53 g
Young men (9–17 years)	57–72 g
Adult women	50 g
Adult men	65 g
During pregnancy	60 g
During lactation	70 g

(Adapted from *Recommendations for Selected Nutrient Intakes of New Zealanders.* Nutrition Advisory Committee, 1983.)

■ ■ ■

For example, a child requires 2 g of protein per kilogram of body weight each day. A 25 kg child (55 lb or 3 st 9 lb) requires 50 g of protein. This can be achieved by eating the following foods in one day:

Food	Protein
2 eggs	12 g
2 bread slices	4 g
600 ml milk	18 g
25 g cheese	7 g
1 potato	3 g
½ cup baked beans	7 g
Total	51 g

■ ■ ■

An adult requires 0.8 g of protein per kilogram of body weight a day. A 60 kg sportswoman (132 lb or 9¼ st) requires 48 g of protein and a 55 kg woman requires 44 g of protein per day. A daily intake of 56 g of protein would meet the needs of a 70 kg sportsman. The main reason for the difference in recommended intakes for children and adults is that adults (except for pregnant women) have finished growing.

■ RECOMMENDED PROTEIN INTAKE FOR SPORTS PARTICIPANTS

Type of sport	Daily intake per kg of body weight
Recreational and casual	0.8 g
Athletes	0.8–1.0 g
Endurance sports	1.0–1.2 g
Weightlifters	1.3–1.6 g
Intense strength sports or training with elevated needs	2–2.2 g

■ ■ ■

■ FOODS PROVIDING 0.8 G PROTEIN PER KG BODY WEIGHT FOR A 70 KG MALE

Food	Serving	Protein g
Cereal	1½ cups	5.0
Skim milk	½ cup	4.5
Fruit juice	½ cup	0.5
Toast	3 slices	6.0
Salad sandwich	4 bread slices	8.0
Chicken	75 g	28.0
Fruit	1 average	0.5
Baked potato	1 average	3.0
Salad/vegetables	1 cup	1.0
	Total	56.5

■ ■ ■

Recommendations for New Zealanders suggest a daily intake of 56 g protein for 70 kg male. Levels of 1–1.5 g per kilogram of body weight have been suggested for most sportspeople. However, some researchers are suggesting that people actively involved in sports, especially endurance activity, may require an increase to 2 g per kilogram of body weight, particularly during the early stages of training. Strenuous bouts of endurance running appear to influence protein metabolism and increase the breakdown of protein tissue (catabolism). The synthesis (build up) of protein appears to be reduced. The following table illustrates the additions to the basic food intake, shown in the previous table, needed to achieve this elevated intake.

53

■ ADDITIONAL FOODS TO PROVIDE 2 G PROTEIN PER KG BODY WEIGHT FOR A 70 KG MALE

Food	Serving	Protein g
Fruit juice	250 ml (1 glass)	1.0
Yoghurt	200 g (1 pottle)	9.5
Cheese	50 g	12.5
Sandwich	2 bread slices	4.0
Fish	150 g	42.0
Baked potato	1 average	3.0
Green peas	½ cup	3.0
Fruit	2 average	1.0
Sandwich	2 bread	4.0
Peanut butter	2 tsp	2.0
Fruit juice	1 glass	1.0
	Total	83.0

■ ■ ■

The basic 56.5 g plus 83 g of additional protein totals 139.5 g. These recommendations show that to provide 2 g per kg of body weight a 70 kg male must consume 140 g of protein. This amount of food can be easily consumed by most males.

Selected reports on sports such as power lifting, and Olympic weightlifting suggest that daily protein intake should be increased to above 2 g per kilogram of body weight for some individuals. Consuming foods only, without the addition of supplements, it is still possible to reach these suggested levels. It is stressed, however, that extremely high levels of training (7-12 hours per day) should accompany these intakes.

■ ADDITIONAL FOODS TO INCREASE PROTEIN INTAKE TO 2.16 G PER KG OF BODY WEIGHT FOR A 70 KG MALE

Food	Serving	Protein g
Ice cream	100 g	4.5
Rice	½ cup	2.0
Fruit	1 cup	1.0
Sandwich	2 bread slices	4.0
	Total	11.5

■ ■ ■

Adding the total (11.5 g) to the previous totals (56.5 and 83) a combined daily intake of 151 g of protein results.

As illustrated, it is easy to obtain this amount of protein from a well-balanced food plan. Most New Zealanders already consume twice the amount of protein required by the body. Protein should make up around 12–15 percent of the energy intake daily and should be supplied by food. Plant protein sources contribute approximately one-third of the protein in the New Zealand diet. Meat (beef) provides over half of the remaining protein. Milk, milk products, fish and eggs all contribute significant amounts.

Contrary to the belief of many coaches, athletes and sportspeople, the protein requirement during heavy exercise is not significantly increased in adults. The amount of protein needed to meet ordinary demands will be sufficient during periods of increased physical activity. This also applies to training with heavy weights which produce increases in muscle mass. However, some initial protein increase may be important in the early phase of training, particularly in weightlifting and intense or strenuous activity.

Protein and exercise

Protein provides energy of 17 kJ per gram, the same as carbohydrate, but the body requires greater effort to convert protein into fuel and it is therefore less efficient as a fuel source. Protein must be converted into a usable form before it can supply energy. This conversion often occurs at the expense of the body tissues. The amino acids are broken down into their basic units (carbon, hydrogen, oxygen and nitrogen) by the liver and the nitrogen is then removed by the kidneys, passing out in the urine.

Consuming excessive quantities of protein (particularly as powders or pills) during performance or training is neither required nor recommended. It may even be contraindicated in many sports as a large protein intake may cause dehydration (protein metabolism requires more water than carbohydrate or fat metabolism) and constipation. Increased water intake is, therefore, encouraged. A gout-like condition has been reported in some susceptible athletes on very high protein diets and this interferes with sports performance.

A high intake of protein increases the loss of potassium, magnesium and calcium (owing to an increase in phosphorus, which causes an imbalance of ratios) and iron. This may be caused by the increased activity of the kidneys. Too much protein may also place an extra burden on the kidneys and liver and become a health concern for some individuals. Consideration must be given to the total energy content of the diet. It is important to remember that protein intake

55

in excess of requirements is stored as fat. Animal sources of protein are higher in fat content than most plant sources, so increasing animal protein in the diet has the potential to increase weight, leading to obesity and the associated risks to health.

A high intake of protein also displaces the percentage of carbo-hydrate in meals, and carbohydrate is the preferred fuel for sports performance. A low carbohydrate/high protein pattern of eating can result in ketosis (an acid condition of the blood usually caused by fasting). Ketones are formed from the incomplete breakdown of fatty acids for fuel. Current recommendations are that intakes of protein should compose 12–15 percent of the total energy intake.

During exercise, the amount of protein available for growth and repair is decreased as protein in the body is broken down and turned over more quickly. However, there is little evidence at present to suggest that increased protein intake for endurance exercise has a benefit for sports performance. Protein provides 1–2 percent of the total energy for exercise. Should exercise be prolonged this can be increased to 5.5 percent.

Some reports indicate that approximately 10 percent of energy can be supplied by protein in carbohydrate-depleted individuals. When glycogen stores are very low or are being used up in exercise, the amino acids may have the potential to provide muscle with fuel for energy, should the exercise be continued. There is some evidence which suggests that particular amino acids, such as leucine, are able to provide this energy during sustained exercise at a faster rate than usual. However, only 4 percent of energy expenditure is provided by protein in carbohydrate-loaded athletes. This reinforces the importance of carbohydrate as the fuel for exercise and activity.

Protein and muscle building

The effect of exercise in stimulating muscle growth has been well documented. To grow, muscle must be worked at 60–80 percent of its maximum capacity. Muscle mass is not directly increased by any addition of high protein foods in the diet. Most of the evidence that protein requirements are increased with exercise programmes comes from studies on endurance exercise. There is an indication from further data that strength training (weight and power lifting) may also elevate protein needs. This provides some scientific support for the belief held by many coaches, athletes, bodybuilders and other sportspeople that there is a benefit to be gained by consuming protein in excess of the Adequate Daily Intake (ADI). The present ADI stands at 65 g for adult men and 50 g for adult women. The ADI takes into account individual variation and a constant level of exercise for the general population. When considering protein levels, it is important to remember that protein intake is not considered insufficient in New Zealand, because we have a high consumption of animal products. The high level of protein in these products is shown in the food intake tables below.

The exact mechanisms for protein use for energy are at present unclear and researchers are still disputing the need for an increased protein requirement for athletes. Studies of cyclists, runners, swimmers and weightlifters have illustrated that when glycogen stores were low more than twice the amount of protein was used for energy compared with high stores of glycogen. The longer the duration of exercise the more protein is used as a source of fuel. Although the amount of energy supplied by protein is small when compared with fat and carbohydrate it remains important for performance. Further research in this area will help to clarify details and provide more information.

It is important to consider the total energy intake of the diet rather than just the protein intake, remembering that carbohydrate spares protein from being used up for energy. It is not necessary to add high protein supplements into the food plan as relatively high intakes

■ PROTEIN CONTENT OF SOME COMMON FOODS

Food	Serving	Protein g
Milk	1 cup	9
Fruit yoghurt	1 × 150 g	6
Cheddar cheese	50 g	12
Cottage cheese	½ cup	17
Ice cream	½ cup	6
Beef	75 g	21
Fish	100 g	25
Egg	1	6
Chicken	75 g	20
Potato	½ cup	2
Corn	½ cup	5
Peas	½ cup	7
Green-leaf veg	½ cup	2-3
Fruit — orange	1 large	1
— avocado	½ small	5
Soya beans	½ cup	14
Bread, wholegrain	2 slices	4

■ ■ ■

of protein can be easily provided from a normal varied baseline eating pattern. Increased energy requirements will generally produce a corresponding natural increase in protein intake sufficient to meet any additional protein requirements. Amino acids supplements add around 2 g protein per day — equivalent to the amount of protein provided by one slice of bread! The major difference is the cost.

7
Salt

New Zealanders eat more than 10 times as much salt (sodium chloride) as they need. Salt intakes have been estimated at 8 g for women and 10 g for men per day. Although salt is essential in the body, the amount needed is very small, about one-tenth of a teaspoon of salt per day. Salt is a compound of sodium and chloride and it is an excess of sodium that can damage health. Table salt contains slightly more than 40 percent sodium. One teaspoon of salt contains over 2 000 mg of sodium. The consumption of two to four teaspoons of salt daily equals 4 400 to 8 800 mg of sodium.

The body requires about 250 mg per day and it has been suggested that intakes of 1 000–3 000 mg are adequate and safe. But for those individuals at risk of high blood pressure an intake of less than 2 000 mg of sodium per day is recommended. This is equivalent to 5 g of salt (one teaspoon), and is easily provided by such foods as meat, milk, eggs and vegetables.

Much salt is added in cooking, at the table, or is hidden in foods such as breakfast cereals, bread, gravy, soups, sauces and flavourings. The salt occurring naturally in foods (for example in cereals) accounts for only 25 percent of our intake. It has been estimated that 25 percent of salt in our diet is added at the table or during cooking, and the greatest contribution to our salt intake (around 50 percent) comes from commercially manufactured foods. These include potato crisps, sausage rolls, snacks, corned beef, soups, sauces and baked products.

As sodium occurs naturally in many foods and this is generally sufficient to meet the active or non-active person's sodium requirements, it is not necessary to add salt.

59

Most people are aware of the salt content of potato chips and roasted peanuts. Other foods high in sodium include baking soda, baking powder, monosodium glutamate (MSG), antacids, Vegemite, Marmite and stocks. Although Vegemite and Marmite are considered high in salt it is important to consider also how much of a particular food is consumed. These two spreads are generally used in small amounts. In fact, there may be more salt in the bread and butter than in the spread added. Three crackers have almost the same amount of salt as one slice of bread. Milk naturally contains sodium. Therefore, milk products, such as yoghurt, will also contain sodium. However, with some milk products, such as cheese, more salt is added during processing.

Sodium and chloride do have important functions in the body, however, and are essential constituents for health. Sodium is needed to maintain water balance in the body. Sodium and chloride not required by the body is excreted in the urine and, of course, some is lost in the sweat. Consuming large amounts of salt requires the kidneys to work quickly to maintain a balance by removing the excess. Reducing the intake of salt limits the amount lost by these two methods and hence the workload on the kidneys. Reducing the intake of salt may also improve calcium status as high intakes cause unavoidable losses of calcium in the urine.

Excessive salt in the diet has been linked with hypertension, or high blood pressure. High blood pressure can result in heart or kidney disease or stroke. In northern Japan, where sodium intakes are over 10 000 mg per day, approximately 40 percent of the population suffer from high blood pressure. In the USA about 20 percent have high blood pressure. A high percentage of the retired population require some form of blood pressure control. In some areas of Africa, New Guinea and South America where the consumption of sodium is very small high blood pressure is almost unknown. In the Solomon Islands two groups of the population used different cooking methods to prepare food. Some of the people living with the group that cooked in seawater developed hypertension. Those living with the other group, where food was cooked in fresh water, were free of the disease. It must also be remembered that individuals vary in their susceptibility to developing hypertension.

Sodium and exercise

The sportsperson has no need to add extra salt to foods as the normal New Zealand eating pattern provides more than an adequate amount to replace those losses due to exercise and perspiration. The use of salt tablets may in fact be harmful to performance and overall health. Salt tablets may cause nausea, vomiting and dizziness, all of which interfere with performance, and may increase the effects of dehydration when insufficient fluid is consumed. Dehydration occurs because the salt draws fluid into the gut rather than allowing it to be absorbed into the bloodstream. Intense exercise lasting for long periods of time may require the addition of salt in the recovery meal, or some sodium may be added for ultra endurance events. But there is no need to add extra salt to meals or fluids before competition or events.

Many symptoms once thought to result from a lack of salt are due to dehydration. An athlete who is dehydrated and consumes a large amount of salt will further dehydrate the tissues. This can be extremely dangerous.

Reports have indicated that some athletes in ultra endurance events (for example, the Ironman in Hawaii), instead of appearing dehydrated after the event, are in fact bloated, with swollen abdomens, puffy hands and swollen ankles. Blood circulation can be affected and mental confusion may result. This depletion of sodium (or water intoxication) occurs when there is a large loss of sodium combined with changes in water balance under intense exercise. Drinking fluids which contain little or no sodium can add to the effect. However, it is important to remember that these are ultra endurance events and water intoxication appears to occur in the less-well-trained athletes. More information is needed before recommendations can be given regarding added salt intake and this is not an excuse to eat high salt foods. Nevertheless, all fluid should be experimented with in training and not left to the day of the race.

If salt intake has been reduced, less sodium will be lost in the sweat; studies have shown that people who reduce salt intake do not suffer any more cramp than they did previously.

Reducing salt intake

To reduce your salt intake, taste food before adding any extra. Many people automatically salt their food before the meal is even tasted and over 1 g of salt can be added this way. Try using pepper or lemon juice instead.

Use only a little salt in the cooking. A microwave is an asset when reducing salt as vegetables cooked in a microwave do not need any added salt. Add flavour by using herbs, spices, lemon juice, grated orange and lemon rind, vinegar, curry powder, mustard, garlic, onions, green peppers, tabasco sauce, chilli and wine. There is an increasing number of low-salt foods or salt-reduced foods appearing on the supermarket shelves. These range from butter and margarine to bread, soups, cheese, breakfast cereals, crackers and seasonings.

Salt is an acquired taste. Many infants develop a taste for salt when solids are introduced which contain added salt. Reduce salt intake gradually. Eat smaller amounts of salty foods less often. Watch out for baking and preserving ingredients which are high in salt. These include sodium bicarbonate (baking soda), baking powder, sodium nitrate, sodium nitrite and sodium-based additives and preservatives. Salt is a common preservative found in many foods. Very salty foods include pickled meats (corned beef), soya sauce, garlic salt, salty snacks (chips etc.). Meat extracts, ham, parmesan cheese, cheese spreads, anchovies, bottled sauces, gravy and other packet sauce powders are all high salt foods. Look for foods with the words 'no added salt' on the label. Buy fresh ingredients where possible. Canned peas are about 250 times as salty as fresh peas.

Reading food labels

Foods which contain less than 150 mg of sodium per serving are very low in sodium. Those with around 250 mg sodium per serving contain moderate levels and foods with sodium content over 250 mg per serving are high. Some examples of foods which are available with no added salt include crackers, cheese, soups, canned fish and canned vegetables.

Foods high in salt

table salt	canned fish
vegetable salts	tuna
garlic salt	salmon
MSG (monosodium glutamate)	sardines
soya sauce	butter
dried stocks	potato chips
gravy powders	salted snacks
caviar	margarine
yeast extracts	takeaways
salted cracker	canned soups
processed meats	pizza
salami	bread
corned beef	hard cheeses
ham	
luncheon sausage	
sausages	

Foods with moderate salt levels

biscuits
salted nuts
canned vegetables
pastry
cake
cereals and muesli
soft cheeses
    cottage cheese
    cream cheese

yoghurt
ice cream
milk
chilli sauce
tomato purée
fresh shellfish
salted peanut butter

Foods low in salt

all fresh fruit
all fresh vegetables*
frozen vegetables*
unprocessed foods*
honey
rice*
eggs*
herbs
dried beans*
pasta*
fresh garlic
onion
vinegar
tea, coffee
cream

mineral waters (check label)
fruit juices
low-salt vegetable juice
puffed cereals
flour
meat*
fish*
chicken*
pork*
bran
'no added salt' foods
whole grains
unsalted butter
low-salt margarine

* Only if cooked in unsalted water.

■ ■ ■

8
Fluids

Next to oxygen, water is the most important substance for human life. A person can only survive five to six days without water. Water is also an important source of minerals. Inadequate water will compromise sports performance, as the participant becomes dehydrated.

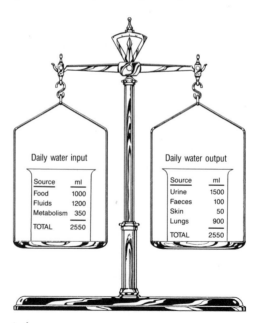

Water balance in humans.

(Adapted from McArdle et al. See bibliography.)

If asked to name the single most important food for physical performance it would have to be water. Water is the one nutrient critical to athletic performance, yet in training and competition it is often neglected. Dehydration hinders performance, interferes with coordination, motivation and concentration, and reduces endurance.

■ PERCENTAGE OF WATER IN SOME TISSUES

49–60% of a person's weight is water
20–25% of fat is water
72% of muscle weight is water

■ ■ ■

These figures vary among individuals. A man is composed of around 55 percent water; 50 percent of a woman is water. Men carry a higher percentage of water because of the extra muscle mass. The 'average' man and 'average' woman contain 42 and 35 litres of water respectively.

Fluids and exercise

Fluid losses of one to two litres per hour are not uncommon during exercise in hot conditions and can exceed three litres in some situations. An athlete can lose 2–4 percent of body weight through sweat and a marathon runner may lose 6–8 percent. A 4 percent loss in a 68 kg (10½ st) man is a loss of 2.7 kg (6 lb), which equals 2 to 3 litres of water. Dehydration occurs with the loss of around 1 percent of body weight. A loss of more than 2 percent in body weight because of dehydration reduces work capacity, leads to a decreased blood volume, increases heart rate, and impairs body temperature control. Any further loss of body water will eventually lead to exhaustion, heat stroke and collapse of the body circulatory system. Death can occur at this stage.

Every living cell in the body requires water to function. Water is essential for blood circulation, removal of waste products, maintaining body temperature control and sweating, and the transport of nutrients. The purpose of sweating is to cool the body through evaporation. When sweat evaporates heat is released from the blood near the skin, which cools the body. As water is lost through perspiration, greater demands are placed on the circulation system. The heart rate increases, the flow of blood to the skin decreases and body temperature rises. The lost water must be replaced or performance is affected.

65

Maintaining fluid balance

To maintain fluid balance you should be fully hydrated prior to your game or event. Drinking large amounts of alcohol the night before the event is not recommended. Fluid should be consumed up to 30 minutes before exercise (about 400–600 ml, depending on the individual). During the game or event small amounts of fluid should be taken often. For example, at each water stop during road races and marathons, or every 10–20 minutes, drink 100–150 ml. Drink regularly during triathlons, in cycle races and during substitution and time-outs in basketball. Do not wait until you are thirsty. Try to organise water breaks wherever possible and drink even if you are not thirsty.

Cold diluted drinks are preferable. Cold drinks empty from the stomach more rapidly than warm drinks and assist in lowering the body's internal temperature. Within 15 minutes of drinking a glass of water two-thirds of this water is absorbed into the circulation system. Because drinks high in sugar take longer to empty from the stomach they are less effective for fluid replacement. These drinks, which take an additional 15 minutes to be absorbed, are not recommended.

Plain water is the best fluid. Unless the activity lasts for more than two hours, water is all that is needed. If fruit juice is used it must be diluted. Commercial fluid replacement drinks are often too concentrated and these should also be diluted. (For more on commercial replacement drinks, see chapter 19.)

Condition the body to get used to taking fluids, particularly during training and practice events or games. Following any period of exercise it is very important to rehydrate immediately to enhance recovery and it may be necessary to supply your own fluid to do this. Record your weight before and after exercise. Replacing around 50 percent of the predicted loss should prevent heat injury and offset any effects on performance.

Splash water on the skin to aid the cooling process. Salt tablets are not recommended. In warmer environments, acclimatise to exercise gradually.

Ways to make water taste great

- Add a few drops of fresh lemon juice or add commercially prepared pure lemon juice.

- Add a few drops, according to taste, of lime juice or lime juice cordial. Check the ingredient list to assess the amount of added sugar. Generally a teaspoon of lime juice cordial per 250 ml of water is sufficient.

- Crush fresh mint leaves (three to four per litre). Peppermint, spearmint, applemint and standard mint work best.

These flavoured drinks can also be frozen into ice cubes and added to water. Make the drink slightly stronger if it is to be frozen as flavoured ice cubes become more diluted when melted.

Keep cold water in the refrigerator covered to avoid absorbing odours from other foods.

Caffeine

Information concerning the effect of caffeine and cola beverages on sports performance remains controversial and inconclusive. Caffeine is found in tea, coffee, cola beverages and products made with cocoa. In excessive amounts it is a banned substance or disqualifying drug. However, limiting the intake of caffeine to a social cup of coffee or cola drink is not considered excessive.

Caffeine is a stimulant to the central nervous system with a widespread effect on the body. It affects the heart and skeletal muscle, and respiration. Its diuretic action, increasing the production of urine, results in further loss of body fluids.

The use of caffeine leads to increases in metabolism, temperature, blood pressure, gastric acid secretion and nervous tension. Loss of hand steadiness, trembling and muscle tension have also been reported as consequences of the consumption of caffeine. Within 30–60 minutes caffeine levels peak in the bloodstream. Long-term use has led to insomnia (inability to sleep), depression, irritated stomach and anxiety. There are also side-effects associated with withdrawal, which include headaches and tiredness. Decaffeinated products are readily available.

Caffeine has been reported as stimulating the use of fat (fatty acids) for fuel by increasing their release into the bloodstream. It is thought that this may spare glycogen and enhance endurance exercise. This effect appears to be dose related and is also dependent on body composition and previous intake of caffeine. A couple of cups of coffee before an event has been shown to enhance endurance and cyclists have improved the amount of strenuous exercise performed. However, this finding is only relevant to continuous exercise lasting over an hour.

Caffeine is a potentially harmful drug and the benefits to performance in sports should be weighed against the risks. Large doses of caffeine in the form of coffee can induce chronic stomach cramps, headaches, irritability and diarrhoea. All these symptoms impair sports

67

performance. Some sportspeople have an allergic reaction to caffeine and associated substances, so it is important to be aware of the caffeine content of foods, medicines and beverages.

■ CAFFEINE CONTENT OF SOME COMMON FOOD

Average serving	Caffeine content
Filtered coffee	115 mg
Percolated coffee	80 mg
Instant coffee	65 mg
Decaffeinated coffee	5 mg
Tea	60 mg
Cocoa drinks	4 mg
Chocolate milk	5 mg
Energy chocolate	20 mg
Chocolate syrup	4 mg
Cola beverages	36–45 mg
Diet cola beverages	36–45 mg

■ ■ ■

Pain relief, cold medicines and diuretics may also contain caffeine. If in doubt, read the label or consult your doctor. Lemonade, ginger ale and soda water are caffeine-free products.

Do not experiment with foods and drinks containing caffeine during crucial events. Well-trained sportspeople are already very efficient in metabolising fatty acids for fuel. Because of the side-effects of caffeine and its labelling as a banned substance it is not recommended. Further research is required.

Alcohol

Drinks containing alcohol are very high in energy (kilojoules) for three reasons. First, alcohol is the second highest source of energy, gram for gram, in the diet after fats; 1 g of alcohol contains 30 kJ. Secondly, the mixers used with alcoholic drinks tend to be high in sugar (soft drinks such as lemonade and cola, and fruit juices). Thirdly, there is a tendency for alcoholic drinks to be included as an extra food item in the eating pattern rather than as part of the overall total intake. Two cans of beer a day for one year would result in an increase of 483 000 kJ (115 000 Cal), or 8 kg (33 lb) in weight. One glass of wine a day for a year adds 420 kJ (100 Cal) per day, or 4.5 kg (10 lb) a year. Provided you use alcohol in moderation a social drink need not be a major hazard to your eating plan.

For the sportsperson, alcohol provides energy; but it also hinders performance for 36–48 hours after consumption if used inappropriately. Therefore, no alcohol should be consumed 48 hours prior to a sports event. Heavy drinkers also tend to consume an inadequate amount of food, resulting in the development of various nutritional deficiencies in the long term. The effects of alcohol on sports performance include early fatigue, poor coordination and impaired concentration. However, if drunk with meals, alcohol may cause no harm after the game or event as long as only small amounts are consumed after adequate hydration.

It is important to remember that alcohol, especially spirits, contains very few nutrients apart from calories, and energy in this form is not utilised by the body for exercise. Try diluting alcoholic drinks with ice, water or fruit juice. Alternate alcoholic beverages with drinks of soda water or fruit juice and slow down the speed with which drinks are consumed. Maintaining adequate hydration is essential for performance. Alcohol has a diuretic action; it causes the body to lose more fluid, which must then be replaced.

■ ALCOHOL AND ENERGY LEVELS COMPARED WITH EXERCISE

Amount of alcohol	kJ	Cal	Activity in minutes Walk	Bike	Swim	Jog
1 small port	672	160	31	25	19	16
1 glass beer	483	115	22	18	14	12
1 nip gin	441	105	20	16	12	11
1 nip whisky	504	120	23	16	14	12
1 glass wine	357	85	16	13	10	9
1 50 ml sherry	357	85	16	13	10	9
1 nip brandy	315	75	14	12	9	8

■ ■ ■

Alcohol taken directly before a game, workout or event will have a direct effect on the central nervous system. Alcohol depresses the brain's ability to make judgements, reduces and hinders fine muscle skills, and slows reaction times and coordination (especially hand/eye coordination, which is important in sports such as golf, tennis, squash, cricket, hockey, netball and archery). Balance is compromised and reflex responses are slowed.

Alcohol is extremely harmful if taken before endurance events. The metabolism of alcohol takes priority once it enters the bloodstream. The alcohol is metabolised before glucose, reducing blood sugar and causing early fatigue during the endurance event. In addition, alcohol disturbs water balance in the body tissues and muscle cells, and promotes dehydration through its diuretic effect.

Nutritional Goals for New Zealanders (see Bibliography) recommends a reduction in alcohol. This does not mean the sportsperson should increase the consumption of low alcohol alternatives such as wine cooler or low alcohol beer. Low alcohol beer provides an alternative for social drinks but is not a substitute for water. They contain less energy and may assist with weight reduction if replacing standard beers, but this is relative to the amount consumed. Should alcohol be consumed before an event, limit to amount to a couple of beers or glasses of wine and drink plenty of water.

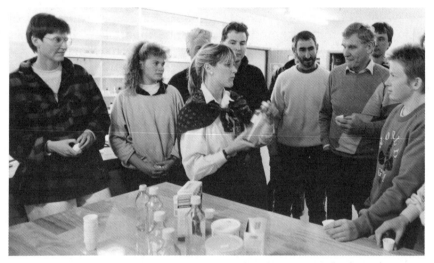

The author discusses the appropriate use of various sports drinks with students in sports nutrition at Waikato Polytechnic.

Remember that water is the best fluid for any event or game lasting under two hours. Endurance and ultra endurance events require special attention. When contemplating glucose solutions as fluids it is important to remember the effects of sugar and insulin on blood glucose levels, which can result in impaired performance. As the carbohydrate content of the drink increases, the time taken for fluid to clear from the stomach is increased. Fluids high in sugar (glucose) decrease the emptying from the stomach leaving a feeling of fullness and reducing fluid absorption. Water taken before, during and after the game will enhance performance by preventing dehydration.

9
Dietary fibre

Mention the word fibre and most people think of oat bran, bran flakes and coarse textured or rough foods. Previously, dietary fibre (the preferred term) was called roughage, denoting the coarse texture of food, but dietary fibre includes many different types of fibre. Once ignored, dietary fibre now features prominently as an important part of a balanced healthy diet. Recent research has shown that the inclusion of various types of dietary fibre in the diet (oatbran and legumes, for instance) is responsible for reducing blood cholesterol levels.

Dietary fibre in itself does not actually lower blood cholesterol levels or stabilise blood sugars. However, because of the function of bran in the digestive tract these benefits have been observed in some people. Dietary fibre affects digestion in three ways. It influences the passage of food through the gut, the absorption of nutrients and the excretion of waste products. However, these effects vary depending on the type of food in which the dietary fibre is present and the other structural components found in the food.

Different types of dietary fibre

Dietary fibre (cellulose, hemicellulose, lignin, pectin and gums) is the part of a food, usually a plant food, that survives digestion, provides bulk in the diet and aids in the functioning of the digestive system. It is found in foods such as fruits, vegetables, wholegrain breads and cereals, dried peas and beans, nuts and seeds. There are three basic types of dietary fibre — cereal dietary fibre (the safest, easiest fibre to add into any eating pattern), dietary fibre from fruits and vegetables, and fibre-related binding agents.

Cereal fibre

Cereal fibre softens and adds bulk to the bowel contents. The major sources are bran, breads and cereals. Inclusion of cereal fibre in the eating pattern eliminates or reduces the problems of straining (which occurs during constipation) that may lead to haemorrhoids (piles) and diverticulitis. Constipation can also be a future indicator of bowel disease. Cereal fibre also reduces the need for laxatives, which, in addition to being expensive, may produce long-term harmful effects if used frequently. Cereal fibres shorten the transit time, which is the time food residue takes to pass through the digestive process. The benefit of this is that it reduces the amount of contact in the bowel of any cancer-causing substances.

Excessive consumption of dietary fibre may lead to diarrhoea, irritation of the gut lining and flatulence and reduce the absorption of nutrients such as minerals. So keep the intake of dietary fibre in balance.

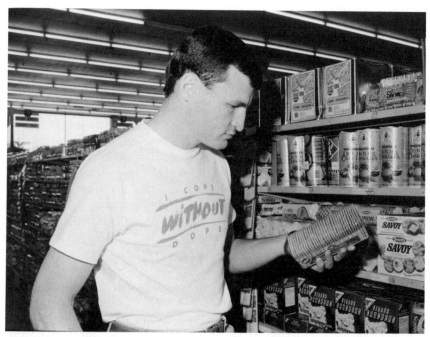

Chris White, of the New Zealand rowing team, checks out nutritional analysis information as he shops.

Fruit and vegetable fibre

Fruit and vegetables contain dietary fibre, pectin and gums, and these have a different action in the bowel from cereal fibres. Pectins, found in high concentrations in apples and orange and lemon pith, slow down the absorption of nutrients. This is one reason diabetics show an improvement in blood sugar control on a high fibre diet. The sugars, particularly glucose, are absorbed more slowly into the bloodstream. Rolled oats and some beans, such as haricot (used in canned baked beans) and kidney (found in bean salads), have been shown to act in a similar manner.

High fibre diets slow down the digestion and absorption of carbohydrates and fats. This provides a lower, longer, more constant supply of energy and avoids the rapid rise in blood glucose levels.

Other fibre

Some fibre-like agents act by binding bile acids and by-products of cholesterol metabolism. Binding makes them unavailable for digestion and absorption resulting in a lowering of total cholesterol. Foods found to contain these substances are legumes (especially soya beans, kidney beans, lentils), peanuts, oats, asparagus and spinach.

Fibre, health and weight control

For good general health it is important to provide adequate fibre in the diet. This can easily be achieved by adding wholegrain varieties of bread and cereals. These include brown rice, wholegrain pasta, oats, oat bran and barley. Use fresh fruits and leave the skins on vegetables where possible. Increase the use of legumes, such as dried peas, beans, lentils, baked beans and split peas. Add nuts and seeds to salads for variety but, as these are high in fat, use them in moderation.

To increase the dietary fibre content of your diet start by adding a couple of small teaspoons of bran flakes (baking bran) into porridge or on cereals and increase this amount gradually. If the level of dietary fibre is increased too rapidly, or too high a volume is used initially, several uncomfortable side-effects may occur. These range from passing excessive amounts of wind, feeling very bloated or distended in the abdomen, diarrhoea or even constipation. It is very important to drink adequate water and other fluids. Remember, everyone has a different tolerance level for dietary fibre.

Body weight can be controlled by adding more foods which are high in dietary fibre to the normal eating pattern. These foods generally contain fewer kilojoules (therefore are lower in energy) and provide more bulk to meals. By adding the extra bulk to meals dietary fibre helps to maintain the feeling of fullness longer and also slows down eating through increasing the amount of time spent chewing. The symptoms of some diseases (constipation and diverticular disease) can be reduced by increasing the dietary fibre content of meals.

Fibre is not a single substance but a mixture of different substances. The type and amount of fibre present varies depending on where the fibre comes from.

■ FIBRE COMPONENTS AND THEIR FUNCTIONS

Type	Food sources	Function
Cellulose	Wheat bran, cereals, seeds, stringy fibre in vegetables, nuts	Effective bulking agent and relieves lower bowel discomfort or constipation.
Hemicellulose	Legumes, lentils, all breads, vegetables, nuts, rice, seeds	Helps to prevent haemorrhoids and diverticular disease
Pectin	Apples, citrus peel, marmalade, jam and fruit	Forms a gel and may assist with reducing blood cholesterol levels
Saponins	Alfalfa, asparagus, chick peas, kidney beans, oats, peas, peanuts, spinach, sunflower seeds	Bind bile acids which are not reabsorbed and the body uses cholesterol to make more acids
Lignin	Potatoes, pears, carrots, woody fibre of cereal husks, root vegetables	Also binds bile acids and reduces cholesterol levels
Gums	Oats, legumes	Role in lowering cholesterol levels. Slow absorption of sugars, assisting blood glucose control
Polysaccharides, legumes, grains		Assists with bulk in bowel

■ ■ ■

Increasing dietary fibre

New Zealanders are encouraged to eat around 30 g of dietary fibre per day. This must be done gradually and, to be effective, must become part of long-term eating patterns. To obtain 10 g of dietary fibre per day you would need to eat one of the foods from the following list each day. As 30 g of dietary fibre per day is the recommended intake, including three selections from the list each day would provide this amount.

■ REQUIRED DIETARY FIBRE FROM SOME FOODS

Wholegrain bread (Fibre content varies depending on variety of bread)	3–4 slices
Mixed grain bread	4–5 slices
Brown bread	6½ slices
White bread	14 slices
Crackers (wholegrain)	6
Cornflakes	500 g (15 cups)
Muesli	½ cup (120 g)
Muesli bars	2–4
Weetbix	5 (70 g)
All Bran	30 g (1 cup)
Bran flakes (cereal)	70 g (2 cups)
Baking bran (unprocessed)	20 g (4 tablespoons)
Brown rice (cooked)	3½ cups
Broccoli	3 cups
Corn	2 large cobs
Tomato	3½ cups
Pumpkin	2 servings
Peas	1 large cup
Potato	2 medium with skin
Cabbage	4 cups
Silverbeet	2½ cups
Dates	¾ cup
Dried apricots	40 g
Fruit salad	1½ cups
Prunes	60 g
Tamarillo	2½
Kiwifruit	3 large
Banana	3 large
Apple	4 large

■ ■ ■

There are some instances where a pattern of eating that includes a high intake of dietary fibre may need to be changed. This appears necessary for endurance (marathons) and ultra-endurance events, when an empty bowel, or one with the minimum of residue, is more comfortable and convenient. A lower dietary fibre intake will need to be followed a few days before the game or event. Use white bread, white rice, cornflakes and rice bubbles. Once the sporting event is over a high dietary fibre intake can be gradually reintroduced.

■ EXAMPLE OF A HIGH FIBRE MENU

Meal	Food Group	Example	Fibre g
Breakfast	3 S* bread & cereal	½ cup muesli	7
	2 whole grain toast	6 slices	
	1 S fruit	1 banana	–
	1 S milk	1 cup trim milk	–
	1 S fat	1 tsp margarine	–
Lunch	4 S bread and cereal	4 wholegrain bread	10–12
	2 S meat	75 g chicken	–
	1 S vegetable	1 cup salad vegetables	4
	1 S fruit	1 nectarine	2
Dinner	2 S meat	75 g beef	–
	3 S vegetables	1½ cups stir-fry veges	6
	2 S cereals	1 cup brown rice	5
	2 S fruit	1 cup fruit salad	6
Snacks	3 S fruit	2 apricots	
		1 pear	4
		2 apples	4
	1 S milk	1 berry yoghurt	1
	2 S cereal	8 wholegrain crackers	11
		TOTAL	60 g
Analysis:	Energy 10.5 MJ	2 500 Cal	
	CHO 418 g	67%	
	Fat 47 g	17%	
	Protein 104 g	16%	

*S = one serving. Replacing wholegrain bread, crackers and brown rice with white varieties reduces the fibre content to 47 g. These products collectively provide 33 g of fibre, their replacements only 10 g.

■ ■ ■

10
Vitamins and minerals

If all the previous recommendations are followed and balanced eating patterns are developed and maintained, there should be no need for any supplementation through the use of vitamin and mineral tablets, powders or drinks. The nutritional aid most commonly abused by athletes is probably vitamin and mineral supplements. Surveys in the United States have shown that three out of four adults believe taking extra vitamins will provide additional energy, regardless of how adequate the diet. However, cases of vitamin poisoning are being reported with increasing frequency.

All groups of the population should rely on consuming a wide selection of foods, rather than taking supplements to reduce the risk of nutritional deficiencies or excesses. However, there are a few groups of sportsmen and sportswomen who may be required to give extra attention to the intakes of particular nutrients.

The groups of sports participants listed below may require extra attention to their food intake, and in some circumstances a supplement may be required:

- Women with excessive menstrual bleeding may need iron.

- Young women during distance training may need iron and possibly calcium.

- Women who are pregnant or breastfeeding may need iron, folic acid and calcium.

- People with a very limited diet, where intakes of all the nutrients are inadequate.

77

- Some vegetarians may not receive adequate calcium, iron, zinc or vitamin B_{12}.

- Certain diseases, disorders or drugs may interfere with nutrient intake, digestion, absorption or excretion.

Excessive doses of some vitamins are known to produce toxic side-effects. If a little is good, more may not necessarily be better, and can in fact be harmful to health and reduce optimum performance. There is no scientific evidence to suggest that sportspeople as a group have an increased need for vitamins as supplements, nor will these improve sports performance.

When considering physical performance and food intake together, energy levels and scientific nutrients become highlighted rather than personal preferences, flavour or the appearance of the food. The function of food becomes one of supplying the body with the essential ingredients to enable an efficient, effective and sometimes powerful and sustained performance in sport.

What are vitamins?

Vitamins are organic compounds or chemicals that are required by the body in varying amounts to enable it to function, grow and develop. Generally, as they are not produced by the body (with the exception of some vitamin K production by the bacteria of the gut), they must be supplied by the food eaten on a regular basis. Vitamins do not provide energy directly themselves but are essential requirements in many of the complex reactions involved in the release of energy. This is particularly true of the B vitamins.

A wide range of vitamins exists. Vitamins B and C are soluble in water and vitamins A, D, E and K are soluble in fat. The vitamin B complex can be further broken down into vitamins B_1 or thiamine, B_2 or riboflavin, B_3 or niacin, folate, B_6 or pyridoxine, and B_{12}. The water-soluble vitamins are not generally stored in the body and are excreted in the urine. This is an area of controversy, as large doses of both vitamin C and B_6 are known to produce side-effects and there is some evidence to suggest that there is some storage by the body. The fat soluble vitamins are stored in the body lipid (fat) tissues and the liver. They are known to be toxic if allowed to accumulate in these tissues.

Some vitamins are converted from other substances (provitamins). For example, vitamin A is produced from carotene, the yellow-orange colour found in fruits and vegetables. Vitamin D can also be metabolised by the action of ultraviolet light on the skin. As mentioned, vitamin K is produced by bacteria in the gut. Niacin (vitamin B_3) can be manufactured from a protein called tryptophan.

Most vitamins are supplied to the body in food such as whole grains, fruits and vegetables. These are excellent sources of most vitamins. However, it is essential to eat a wide variety of foods to obtain all the vitamins. Milk and milk products contain good sources of riboflavin (vitamin B_2), and meat, especially lean pork, is a good source of thiamine (vitamin B_1). Bread and yeast products are excellent sources of all the B vitamins (especially the wholemeal and wholegrain cereals).

Unfortunately, the misconception that vitamins supply energy directly to the body and additional vitamins, therefore, improve physical performance remains a common belief among many sportspeople. This theme has been used to promote supplementation. Deficiencies may occur when moving abruptly from a higher dose (using a supplement) to a lower dose (stopping supplements) of vitamins. This appears more common in particular vitamins, especially vitamin C. In New Zealand today, clinical vitamin deficiencies are rare, and, in the future, problems of vitamin toxicity may become more common.

Role of vitamins in sports performance

Vitamins are involved in various complicated functions in the body. They play an important role in ensuring healthy eyes, bone growth, healthy skin and teeth, wound healing, the formation of red blood cells, energy release (the metabolism of proteins, carbohydrates and fats), and the production of a large number of enzymes and chemical processes in the body. The deficiency of certain vitamins may impair physical performance, particularly those vitamins with functions associated with energy production.

Most of the water-soluble vitamins are involved with enzymes or processes essential to fat and carbohydrate metabolism. They do not provide energy themselves but perform important functions in the energy pathway. The inter-relationship between the vitamins themselves and other nutrients is still a major field of investigation, and some of the answers remain unclear, unknown or controversial.

A study performed on male runners over nine months compared the use of a vitamin supplement with a placebo. Various tests were performed examining exercise performance. No improvement was found and it appears that sportsmen and sportswomen consuming a well-balanced diet do not require vitamin or mineral supplements.

See appendix 1.

Minerals

It is important to remember that large doses of some minerals can be hazardous to the body, performance and health in general. Soil in New Zealand has low levels of some minerals, including iron, zinc, copper, iodine, selenium and fluorine. However, there is no evidence of wide-scale deficiencies of these minerals among the general population. The most common nutritional deficiency reported in athletes and sportspeople is iron deficiency.

Minerals are inorganic (non-living) elements that include metals (iron, calcium, sodium, potassium, magnesium, zinc) and non-metals (chlorine, iodine, sulphur and phosphorus). Minerals are classified as macronutrients (the body requires more than 100 mg per day) or micronutrients (the body requires trace amounts or only a few milligrams per day). Minerals make up 4-6 percent of the sportsperson's weight. For a 58 kg woman minerals make up approximately 2.7 kg of her weight; the portion of minerals in a 70 kg male is around 4 kg. Some minerals can be toxic if intakes are excessive. However, this is unlikely to happen through food intakes, except in some rare disease states or through cooking methods. For example, cooking in copper pots, using copper teapots, or drinking water from copper pipes.

Minerals are essential to the body and we are unable to survive without them, but they are required in very small quantities and often work with the vitamins in body structures. For example: zinc works with vitamin A in tissue repair, magnesium with vitamin B_6 in protein synthesis, selenium with vitamin E as antioxidants, calcium and phosphorus with vitamin D for bone formation, and cobalt is important in the formation of vitamin B_{12}.

Mineral deficiencies

Minerals are not destroyed by heat. Although severe deficiencies are uncommon, deficiencies can occur when minerals are lost in water (sodium, potassium, chlorine, phosphate, iodine, fluorine and selenium) or excreted in the urine, when foods are refined, or with health problems resulting in poor absorption into the body.

The absorption of some minerals is low; for example, only 10 percent of iron ingested through the mouth is absorbed; zinc absorption is influenced by the amount of fibre (phytic acid) present; rhubarb causes the calcium in milk to be unavailable, and eating large amounts of licorice causes the kidneys to hold onto sodium (salt) and excrete more potassium in the urine, which can affect the heart.

With the exception of iron, calcium and phosphorus, minerals cannot be stored in the body long term as they are excreted daily and used in a number of body processes. Ensuring an adequate supply of minerals on a regular basis becomes important for sportspeople because of the interaction of the minerals with the vitamins, to obtain energy from food.

Our knowledge of the role of minerals in human nutrition is incomplete. Many trace elements are difficult to research as the requirements are so small, and deficiencies are rare and hard to identify.

Role of minerals in sports performance

Many vitamins and minerals interact and work closely together in the body, affecting growth, metabolism and health. A deficiency of one may interfere with the performance or function of another. Some minerals require special attention. (The importance of iron and calcium in sports performance and in general health is discussed further in chapter 12.)

Athletes limiting their energy intake to maintain or reduce weight (gymnasts, dancers, skaters, jockeys and wrestlers, for example) may have lower vitamin and mineral intakes. A daily multivitamin and mineral supplement may be advised for these individuals. These sportspeople should also be encouraged to consume more nutrient-dense foods containing fewer kilojoules. Supplementation is not an excuse to eat a poor diet.

See appendix 2.

Potassium toxicity

One mineral that can cause serious side-effects if taken inappropriately is potassium. Potassium is lost through sweat. Exercising vigorously may cause a deficiency of this mineral, although this occurs only under extreme conditions. Large losses can also occur with considerable loss of water, such as with the use of diuretics (fluid tablets) or laxatives. It is also possible to lose large amounts of potassium through vomiting, or excessive sweating in steam rooms. Potassium deficiencies affect the muscle, causing muscle weakness, diarrhoea and discomfort of the digestive tract. However, a well-balanced diet provides sufficient amounts of potassium without the need for supplements.

Potassium as a supplement has been used by bodybuilders to induce a measured amount of dehydration in an attempt to create greater muscle definition. This substance is potentially dangerous and overuse can be fatal. In the USA, accidental overdoses of potassium salts are known to have caused several deaths in otherwise healthy individuals.

Excessive vitamin intake

Vitamin toxicity is a relatively new phenomenon. The first evidence came from Arctic explorers who, when near starvation, were forced to eat polar bear and dog livers. These two foods are extremely high in vitamin A. This resulted in the explorers' losing their hair, and caused diarrhoea, headaches and sleep problems, leading to their eventual deaths.

There is no evidence to suggest that athletes or sportspeople require additional vitamins. Laboratory tests on blood, urine or tissue samples are available, which detect vitamin depletion from body stores. Iron is the only element that may require some additional consumption. This is important for females active in sport, endurance runners of both sexes and adolescents, especially young females. These athletes require an additional intake because of growth or blood losses and nutritional counselling should be sought in these cases.

Sports participants generally consume vitamins in excess of the adequate daily requirement. Those vitamins often taken in excess include vitamins B, C and E. The issue of vitamin supplementation is under considerable debate. Evidence to date has failed to show any significant improvement in physical performance and recovery rates to warrant recommending their use. There is no direct evidence that exercise results in any increase, destruction or metabolism of the vitamins. A varied diet, involving a wide selection of foods, that meets the increased energy demands of training and competition will result in an adequate intake.

Several studies have shown that between 10 and 70 percent of athletes have abnormal thiamine, riboflavin and pyridoxine values. The questions that concern the athlete, coach, trainer, parent or specialist are: Is the athlete consuming a balanced diet to avoid these abnormal values? Does this actually impair physical performance? Vitamins A and C have not been shown to affect endurance capacity. However, the other water-soluble vitamins may be of concern.

It has been suggested by some researchers that there may be an increase in the body's use of B vitamins with hard training or exercise. This refers to the link between the B vitamins and energy pathways. Thiamine is directly involved with the generation of energy and the requirement for this vitamin is expressed as a function of the energy consumed(usually per 4 200 kJ). Although several studies have shown there is no adverse effect on physical performance in a thiamine deficient diet, a rapid improvement has been noted on these deficient intakes when foods that are high in thiamine (not supplement) have been added to the diet.

It has been suggested that an increase in riboflavin may be required for young women with an increased energy expenditure. This is easily achieved through consuming more milk and cheese (low fat varieties).

Vitamin C, also known as ascorbic acid, is commonly believed to be a protection against a number of illnesses, including the common cold, but much of the evidence is controversial. Studies have implied that additional vitamin C may improve heat tolerance in African miners, but there was no mention of any improvement in health or performance. No improvement in heat tolerance was reported when vitamin C was given to a group of well-fed Americans. This suggests the diet of the Africans may have been marginally deficient and an increase in vitamin C may, in this case, have been appropriate.

A considerable time needs to elapse on a restricted intake before any impairment because of clinical vitamin deficiency can be seen. The risk to sports participants is minimal provided they consume a balanced diet, select a wide range of food and eat sufficient energy foods to meet the needs and demands of training and competition. High energy expenditure sports may require additional B vitamins, which are easily incorporated into the diet by increasing wholegrain cereals. Vitamins and mineral supplements are no substitute for training.

As shown in the tables in appendix 1 and 2, excessive intakes of certain vitamins and minerals can be hazardous to sports performance and may even cause toxic symptoms. Those vitamins

■ EXAMPLES OF VITAMIN TOXICITY

Athlete	Symptoms	Cause
Gymnast	Tingling in neck and back, unsteady movements.	Taking large doses of B6 for premenstrual tension.
Bodybuilder	Skin breaks out in red rash which is very itchy.	Taking large doses of B6 to reduce body water and weight.
Marathon runner	Muscle and joint soreness, headaches, dry skin.	Consuming high intake of vitamin A in multivitamin supplements.
Netballer	Constipation and black stools.	Taking large doses of iron supplements to prevent sports anaemia.
Rower	Nausea and light diarrhoea.	Consuming excessive quantities of vitamin C (5600 times ADI).

■ ■ ■

generally associated with toxic symptoms include: vitamin A, C, B$_6$, and E. The table at the bottom of the previous page shows examples of vitamin overdoses suffered by particular sportspeople.

Vitamin A is toxic at only five times the ADI. Yet supplements containing this amount are available and not uncommon. Toxicity also depends on the type of vitamin A. The vitamin table (see appendix 1) identifies two forms of vitamin A — the animal form (retinol) and a plant form (carotene). Retinol is the form that causes the toxic symptoms. Intakes of carotene cause a harmless yellow-orange colouring of the skin. This can be seen in vegetarians who eat large amounts of carrots and drink carrot and green vegetable juices.

Vitamin D consumed in large amounts can be very serious. Toxic effects have been seen when two and a half times the ADI have been consumed. These include damage to soft tissues, demineralisation (loss of minerals) in bone and damage to the kidneys and arteries. There is no need for New Zealanders to take this vitamin in the form of a supplement as sufficient is provided in the diet and through the action of sun on the skin.

Both vitamins A and D are fat-soluble vitamins, which means they are stored in the body. Toxicity associated with these vitamins is well known. However, overdoses with water-soluble vitamins, although rare, can also occur, and the severity varies among individuals. Remember, the longer the supplement is taken and the higher the dose, the greater the potential for toxic symptoms to occur.

Vitamin B$_6$ is known to cause damage to nerve function if taken in excessive amounts. In one case study, vitamin B$_6$ caused severe migraines when four times the ADI was consumed for stress. Niacin (vitamin B$_3$) toxicity was reported in two American rowers, who experienced discomfort and flushing after taking multivitamin supplements that contained 500 mg of niacin. Skin flushing with severe itching and headaches were reported in people taking as little as 100 mg of niacin per day. The ADI for niacin is 18 mg and minimum safe intake (MSI) is only 5 mg per day.

It has been suggested that the vitamin C requirement could be increased for marathon runners and for other trauma sports, to assist with reducing long-term muscle fibre damage. But supplementation with additional vitamin C is a controversial topic. Athletes should aim to achieve any increased requirement through food. The effects of an overdose of vitamin C include acidosis (changes in the body's chemical balance to a more acid state), kidney stones, gastrointestinal disturbances (usually diarrhoea), destruction of vitamin B$_{12}$, and nausea. Information to date suggests the effects of vitamin C toxicity outweight any benefits of supplementation at levels of 1 g (1 000 mg) per day.

With the above exceptions, much of the evidence available at present indicates that most vitamins are relatively non-toxic. However, more research is needed. It is unwise to assume unlimited amounts of water-soluble vitamins will do no harm. There is the possibility of interaction by these vitamins among themselves and with other nutrients. For example, vitamin E in very large doses has been reported to interfere with the absorption of vitamins A, C and K; it may also cause some minor gastrointestinal upsets.

Among the reasons people involved in sporting activities take vitamin and mineral supplements is to prevent illness — as a form of insurance. But this can prove very expensive as any extra intake of the water-soluble vitamins will be lost in the urine. Other reasons sportspeople consume supplements are as a self-prescribed medicine or tonic, or in the hope of enhancing performance in some way. Because of the volume of food sportspeople generally consume they are at a low risk of suffering any ill-effects from vitamin and mineral deficiencies. More concern is expressed over an excess of these nutrients as supplements in addition to those supplied through food. Do not become susceptible to the claims of manufacturers. If in doubt, seek professional advice.

How to get adequate vitamins and minerals

- Eat a wide selection of foods.

- Retain vitamins in food. Some vitamins (vitamins B and C) are readily destroyed by cooking, others by sunlight (riboflavin) or exposure to oxygen (vitamins C and E).

- Exercise regularly so more food can be eaten to increase selection and variety.

- Keep in mind the effects of age, alcohol, medication, pregnancy, fad diets and poor eating patterns.

- Place more emphasis on nutrient-dense foods. These foods supply more nutrients per serving than other foods.

- Use vitamin and mineral supplements only when a food solution cannot be found — for example, in cases of food allergy, food aversion or food intolerance.

The adequate daily intake recommendations have a safety level built in. Only the minimum safe intake (MSI) indicates the minimal intake to prevent disease. In other countries around the world, such as Australia, the United States and Britain, the recommended daily intake (RDI) is set two to three times higher than the level required to prevent nutrient deficiencies. This allows for individual variation, poor food storage and poor maintenance of body stores. There should be no need for supplements in a pattern of eating that contains adequate energy, wholegrain cereals, low-fat dairy products, lean meat and plenty of fresh fruit and vegetables.

11
Food for specific sports

When information on sportspeople's nutritional status is evaluated, the following factors must be assessed:

- daily energy intakes;

- composition of the diet in terms of the percentage of energy supplied by protein, fat and carbohydrate;

- individual preferences, which influence the foods selected regularly;

- whether there is inadequate intake of specific nutrients, and possible deficiencies or excesses;

- health factors (such as the risk of heart disease or presence of diabetes).

Although athletes generally appear to consume more energy than non-athletes there is a wide range of energy requirements, depending on the individual and the activity in which he or she is involved. Body size and the amount of time devoted to training will influence the amount of food eaten and the total energy required. Some marathon runners and cyclists expend over 8.4 MJ (2 000 Cal) per day in training, and some football players consume 42-58 MJ (10 000-14 000 Cal) per day. Very low energy consumers (33-5 kJ) include gymnasts, dancers and wrestlers competing in weight classes lower than their natural body weight.

It is important that eating patterns do not cause additional stress and concern and that they are suited to the individual sportspeople. Eating can easily be tailored to training schedules. No two people enjoy the same food or types of foods. Allowances must be made for differences in religion, culture, ethnic background and the seasons, as well as personal preferences.

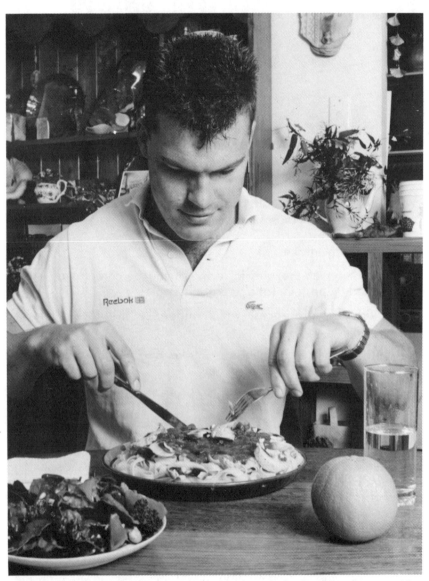

Hammer thrower Phil Jensen requires a high carbohydrate lunch to provide fuel for the evening workout.

Aerobics

While attending class recently I overheard two women discussing what they had eaten before coming to class. One had not eaten all day and the other had just finished a candy bar to provide her with an energy boost. Both left the class before it was half-way through.

For 1 hour's activity, such as an aerobics class, any food eaten just before exercise will not have had time to be digested. Foods high in sugar can even be harmful, causing low blood sugars, nausea and stomach cramps. By not eating any food all day the body glycogen reserves have been depleted, leaving very little fuel for activity.

Eating a high carbohydrate lunch followed by a light snack 3 hours before the class will provide sufficient fuel for a great workout. The class will also be fun and enjoyable rather than a grind. Drink sufficient fluids before, during and after the class.

Athletics

There is a wide range of energy demands for different forms of athletics, depending on the distance run. Each individual athlete must prepare specifically for their event. Sprinters have different requirements from distance athletes. Strength athletes must ensure that weight gain does not result in an increase in their percentage of body fat.

Replacing fuel and glycogen stores after training, particularly after a high intensity session, enables the athlete to get the maximum benefit from the next training session. Fluids are critical. Carbohydrate loading is only a consideration for endurance events lasting longer than 90 minutes. It has several disadvantages for the sprinter because of the excess weight carried, from an increase in body water, and increased stiffness in the muscles.

Basketball, netball, field and ice hockey, soccer

Team events have special sets of problems. Some players need to gain weight and others may have difficulty maintaining weight.

Competitive basketball games are often played in the evening, so a light pre-game meal about 3 hours before should be fine. Plenty of fluids should be encouraged before, during and after. Individual water bottles will help to monitor fluid intake. If training sessions are to be conducted on the day of a game (in the morning), high carbohydrate meals must be organised to replace glycogen levels before the game commences in the afternoon. This is relevant for all sports, particularly those in which participants train, rather than rest, during the 24 hours before a game.

Weight and eating patterns should be monitored during the off-season so that sportsmen and sportswomen are in reasonable condition during pre-season training. As this is when team players are selected, athletes who are fit and healthy have an advantage.

Cricket

Regardless of their position on the field, all players should follow the baseline eating patterns for good health. Even wicketkeepers are required to run at some point in the match. Eating high fat foods has possible long-term disadvantages for heart health. Fluids are important and players should be well hydrated before walking onto the pitch. Bowlers particularly must monitor hydration. Cricketers who carry excess weight expend more energy to move, run, walk or sprint and this can influence endurance over several days of cricket.

Endurance events

At the 25th anniversary of the Fletcher's marathon I observed some disturbing methods being used by runners to maintain their energy levels in the later stages of the race. Two men were seen running while drinking beer, several people ate blocks of chocolate, candy bars, boxes of barley sugars or peppermints during the run. One study of the food intake of Australian marathon runners reported that although some of these elite athletes achieve the recommended levels of carbohydrate intake, many do not.

For success in any endurance activity, whether it be tramping, marathons, triathlons, mountaineering, cross-country skiing or long distance cycling, training is critical and fuelling the working muscles to capacity with glycogen can delay fatigue. For a race taking longer than 3 hours to complete, such as the marathon, light snacks may help, but fluid is the most important factor. For long events, for example the Ironman or the Coast-to-coast run, solid food, liquid meals (such as Ensure) and sports drinks can all play a part. Schedule your food and liquid stops and monitor intake so that nothing is left to chance. For triathlons and distance cycling it is important to begin eating earlier than usual to allow for slow digestion times. Triathletes should begin eating as soon as the cycle phase begins.

Practise the technique of eating and experiment with food during training sessions to reduce the possibility of side-effects. This is particularly relevant to carbohydrate loading, which is not well tolerated by some people. Do not attempt anything new on the day. Stick to what you know and are comfortable with.

Golf

Though golf is not a high intensity sport, it does require endurance as participants will be active for most of the day. Light snacks, adequate fluids and no alcohol are the major nutritional recommendations. Golf requires skill and concentration so if you are sensitive to caffeine, monitor intakes and remember that caffeine also has a diuretic action. There is no need to carbohydrate load for this event.

Gymnastics, wrestling, dance, horseracing (jockeys)

Maintaining a suitable weight is important for peak performance in these activities. Excess weight can be a serious disadvantage. Using drastic methods for rapid weight reduction, such as fasting, semi-starvation, vomiting or laxative abuse, must be avoided. Many of these methods leave the athlete severely dehydrated. Performance is seriously affected and health is often placed at risk if these methods continue. Achieving weight loss within a sensible time frame and setting realistic goals for each individual are important.

Martial arts, boxing

These sports both have the same basic requirements. Often, weight must be gained or lost to enable these sportspeople to compete within a particular weight class. Body fat levels are often lower than for many other sports and weight must be maintained at the appropriate level. Wide fluctuations in weight do not allow for the development of full potential during training.

Carbohydrate loading is not necessary as bouts last an average of only 2–3 minutes. Carbohydrate loading can in fact be a disadvantage as it causes the muscles to feel heavy and stiff. For competitions involving a knockout or for round-robin playoffs it is important to maintain fluids. Eat light snacks if sufficient time is provided between bouts of activity.

Rowing

The nutritional requirements for competition rowing depend on the rower's weight class. Lightweight rowers should maintain weight or be close to their competitive weight before competition. Wide swings in weight should be avoided.

During heavy training or workouts high carbohydrate snacks with plenty of fluids should be provided to replace the glycogen in muscles which is burned as energy. Liquid meals assist those who suffer with nerves and are unable to hold down solid food. These should be consumed at least 3 hours before a race to allow for a slower digestion time. Iron is an important consideration, especially for women rowers.

Rugby, rugby league

Two sports in New Zealand that have received considerable attention in recent years are rugby and rugby league. The requirements for both sports are similar but vary according to the positions played. Each position on the field has its own individual set of characteristics. Some players must gain weight for strength and others may be required to reduce weight for speed.

The pre-game meal depends on the time of the game. Generally this should be eaten at least 3 hours before, and should be a high carbohydrate, low fat meal with sufficient fluids and no alcohol. Gone are the days of a pint with steak and eggs. Fluids should be consumed whenever possible throughout the game and at half-time. Water is the most suitable fluid. Save the sports drinks until after the game and use them as part of the recovery phase.

During the off-season, many players gain weight in the form of increased percentages of body fat. This must then be lost before the new season commences. Maintaining some activity during the off-season and reducing food intake can help to prevent undesirable weight gain.

Skiing

Hydration during events is important. There is a tendency for snow skiers to consume several servings of high fat foods (cream soups, chocolate, rich cocoa drinks and roasted peanuts) and foods high in sugar (candy, barley sugar and muesli bars) for quick bursts of energy. Fat takes several hours to be digested while foods with high sugar contents may induce a hypoglycaemic effect in sensitive people. Aim for high carbohydrate foods with adequate fluids.

Squash

Squash requires speed and skill in addition to concentration, coord- ination and endurance. A player who has neglected to pay attention to his or her diet cannot expect to perform at peak capacity. Fluids are essential and eating during tournaments must be planned. Many sports clubs contract out the catering for these events and the food provided is often high in fat and salt, low in carbohydrate and limited in variety. Most fluids are high in sugar. Pies and toasted sandwiches are favourites, but these do not provide the fuel for peak performance.

Be prepared and pack the athlete's travel kit. This should include a water bottle, fruit juice (to be diluted), crackers, dried fruit, sandwiches or filled rolls, yoghurt and fresh fruit. Leave nothing to chance.

Swimming

Many swimmers train all year round and are often growing adoles- cents with large appetites. One of the problems with swimming training is timing. Many swimmers head off to the pool in the early hours of the morning and often miss breakfast. If it can be tolerated, a light meal of fruit juice, toast, cereal, stewed fruit or muffins should be eaten. However, if breakfast is missed it is important that the body is refuelled. Eating a high carbohydrate breakfast or morning tea, replacing fluid losses and having a high carbohydrate lunch are essential. High quality nutrient dense snacks are important. Swimmers often train twice a day so replacing energy for the afternoon session is critical.

Some swimmers have attempted to use liquid meals before events or training. These still need to be taken 3 hours before the activity to allow time for digestion and are more appropriate after the event or training to replace the glycogen burned for fuel. During periods of intense training (interval training or distance swimming), a liquid meal that is high in carbohydrates can often be an advantage, especially as appetite often diminishes after the activity.

Tennis

The game of tennis often involves long tournaments, sometimes lasting several days in hot weather. Maintaining good hydration is very important. It is essential to follow the baseline patterns with increased carbohydrates (60-65 percent) to maintain glycogen stores. If the tournament lasts longer than 3 hours of continuous play a lightly sweetened beverage such as diluted fruit juice or very diluted sports drinks may be an advantage. These should be tested during training. For meals between games, a light snack of sandwiches, crackers, fruit and plain biscuits is appropriate. The size of the meal will be determined by the length of the break between games. Fluid is the most important consideration.

12
Training meals

No one would consider putting inferior or low-grade petrol into their car. Nor would they let the engine overheat with a dry radiator, or forget to check the oil or the water in the battery. Yet we constantly forget to check on the fuel for the body. Many times meals are missed or lower-grade fuel, such as candy or high fat snacks, is used. Often fluids are drunk only when the body demands them by initiating thirst. And some sportspeople rely on supplements when they feel their battery is run down.

It is generally agreed that a pattern of eating that is high in carbohydrates (55-60 percent), with a corresponding decrease in protein and fat, is the preferred diet for training. Yet many athletes still fail to maintain energy levels. There are many reasons for this, including insufficient knowledge of food, difficulties in food purchase and preparation, limited food preferences, lifestyle, training schedules, and travel and practice times. These factors must be taken into consideration when advising athletes on training diets.

If insufficient carbohydrate is consumed over successive days of training, a progressive depletion of glycogen stores occurs. Feeling tired and lethargic, difficulty in coping with light exercise, and heavy muscles can result from insufficient glycogen replacement in the muscle. (See chapter 20.)

The meals eaten during training can influence overall performance in sports events. Once the baseline eating patterns have been established, training meals require further attention to allow sports participants to get the best out of their training sessions and to recover more effectively.

It is essential to meet the extra energy output during training with an increase in energy input. This is important if weight is to remain stable. Weight gain (increasing muscle mass) and weight loss (decreasing body fat) can also be achieved and the problems of fad diets addressed during the training period.

Iron and calcium require special attention as sports anaemia may appear during periods of intense activity or at the onset of training. Vegetarian eating patterns also need special attention and this is the most appropriate time to experiment with different fluids and other foods that may be taken before or during competition. A sudden change in diet or eating patterns immediately before an important event or competition can have adverse results and be hazardous to sports performance. Remember, no food will make up for deficiencies in training and there are no magic foods or formulas. Without a doubt, after natural ability and dedication to training, nutrition is the factor that most influences sports performance.

For discussion on the effects of sugar and glucose on exercise and sports performance, see chapter 4.

Iron losses and sports anaemia

Investigations to date reveal evidence that suggests iron deficiency is very common among some groups of athletes. Indeed, one Waikato netball team revealed low iron status in 7 out of 10 players. These studies suggested that many sportswomen become prone to iron deficiency, as do both men and women involved in heavy training, especially endurance runners.

Sports anaemia has been described as a result of increased destruction of blood cells, low haemoglobin levels and the stress of exercise. Another possible cause is inadequate protein intakes in the early stages of training. It has been suggested that increasing the protein content could prevent the type of sports anaemia that occurs with high levels of exercise. This is called exercise-induced anaemia. Changes in iron status are usually seen at the start of training and rarely result in clinical anaemia. The body does recover as it adjusts to the metabolic changes of training. In exercise-induced anaemia the iron stores may be depleted without obvious anaemia. It is unclear if depletion is due to inadequate intake, the effect of the exercise, or a combination of both.

Sports anaemia has also been reported in individuals who engage in sports that cause trauma, such as American football and boxing. Iron supplementation would appear essential in these individuals, but

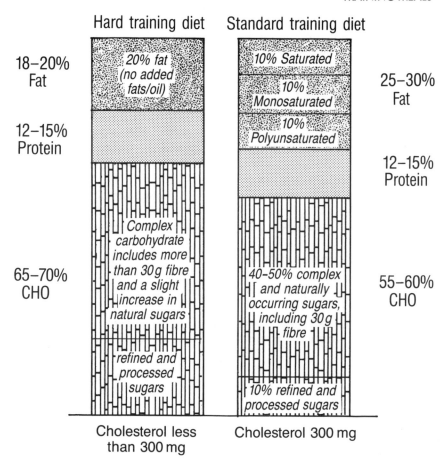

Hard training diet

Standard training diet

18–20% Fat

12–15% Protein

65–70% CHO

25–30% Fat

12–15% Protein

55–60% CHO

20% fat (no added fats/oil)

10% Saturated

10% Monosaturated

10% Polyunsaturated

Complex carbohydrate includes more than 30g fibre and a slight increase in natural sugars

40–50% complex and naturally occurring sugars, including 30 g fibre

refined and processed sugars

10% refined and processed sugars

Cholesterol less than 300 mg

Cholesterol 300 mg

Dietary goals for sportspeople during training.

only after thorough medical investigation. Researchers have considered it inappropriate to recommend regular iron supplementation for those athletes who are not at risk of developing anaemia. All other forms of anaemia must be excluded.

Iron is lost through cells in the gut, skin, hair and a small amount with the bile in the small bowel; the total loss is about 1 mg per day. The body's basic requirement of iron is only 1 mg, but the absorption of iron is extremely inefficient (only 10–20 percent of intake). Iron losses for women are greater (5–45 mg) through menstruation. An additional 1 mg of iron must be absorbed to replace iron lost from one menstrual period. Therefore, iron intake for women should be around 12 mg. The requirement for adult men is 10 mg.

97

Growth also demands more iron. Adolescent females are more likely to be deficient and adolescent males have a large increase in lean tissue, which requires additional iron. Pregnancy also increases the requirement for iron. Regular monitoring of iron status is recommended for optimum performance and sporting ability.

Anaemia is undesirable for athletes as iron plays an important role in energy production. A healthy adult carries about 3–5 g of iron in the body. Iron is essential for haemoglobin (the protein that transports oxygen from the lungs to the muscles), muscle and several enzymes. Iron is involved in many metabolic pathways. It transports oxygen and carbon dioxide and is involved in the respiration of the cells. Low iron levels reduce the supply of oxygen to the muscle and this affects the energy levels as less oxygen is available for energy production. Anaemic sportspeople tire easily regardless of their level of fitness.

About 30–40 percent of iron is in storage and the rest is called working iron. Storage iron is found in the liver, bone marrow and spleen. The following factors contribute to the decrease of iron stores:

- Normal or abnormal blood loss: abnormal losses include blood donation, upper intestinal tract bleeding and heavy menstrual bleeding.

- Inadequate nutrition: poorly planned vegetarian eating or unbalanced food intake over a period of time.

- Poor absorption from the gut and increased loss associated with heavy sweating.

- Losses in the urine.

- Destruction of red blood cells.

Low iron levels impair aerobic endurance. Therefore, replacing or restoring iron status can be beneficial in those athletes who are anaemic. Iron deficiency anaemia decreases work capacity by influencing oxygen uptake and muscle metabolism. Hence during exercise the heart finds it difficult to pump the required amount of blood.

The body is generally able to increase iron absorption when body stores become depleted. However, in long distance runners who are already iron deficient, iron absorption appears to be decreased (usually to about half the level of the non-active iron-deficient individual). It has been suggested that hard physical training may in some way impair the normal absorption mechanism.

The iron stores of a group of female hockey players were monitored over three seasons and a progressive decrease was reported, which implies that long-term sports anaemia may be related to iron deficiency. Assessing haemoglobin and serum ferritin (storage iron) levels will provide a clearer picture.

Groups at risk

Females involved in sport and exercise Regular menstrual losses increase the need for iron. The consumption of a low calorie diet increases the risk as these diets are also low in iron. Intakes of less than 8.4 MJ are often associated with iron deficiency. Female athletes involved in sports such as gymnastics, ballet and distance running, to whom low body fat is an asset, are especially at risk.

Teenage sportsmen A young, growing sportsman has a large in- crease in total haemoglobin and cells owing to increased lean tissue. Therefore, the adequate daily intake (ADI) of iron increases. Reduced iron stores should be suspected if there is a decline in performance. Special consideration must be given to a teenager competing in endurance events.

■ FOODS HIGH IN IRON

Food	Quantity	Iron content mg
Liver	75 g	10.5
Lamb kidneys	75 g	8.5
Dried apricots	½ cup	5.5
Prunes	½ cup	5.5
Dates	½ cup	4.8
Oysters	75 g	4.3
Pork	75 g	4.2
Beef	75 g	3.5
Beans (cooked)	½ cup	2.8
Raisins	½ cup	2.5
Lamb	75 g	2.3
Sardines in oil	5	2.2
Figs	½ cup	2.2
Spinach	½ cup	2.0
Peas	½ cup	2.0
Porridge	1 cup	1.9
Chicken	75 g	1.6
Egg	1	1.2
Baked fish	75 g	1.0
Weetbix	1	0.8
Bread (wholemeal)	1 slice	0.8
Brewer's yeast	1 tsp	0.5

■ ■ ■

Sportspeople who do not eat red meat (semi-vegetarians, strict vegans and those with very low cholesterol eating patterns) Meat is one of the best sources of iron. Non-animal sources include beans, enriched cereals and green vegetables. However, iron from plant sources is not as well absorbed (only 10 percent) as that from animal sources (10–37 percent).

Endurance athletes Perspiration can account for a loss of an additional 1 mg per day of iron for those involved in hard training with heavy sweating. Iron is also lost through the skin, hair, urine and faeces. Inadequate dietary intake, such as sometimes occurs with endurance athletes on restrictive weight reduction diets, creates further risks to iron status.

To reduce the risk of iron deficiency anaemia:

- Use a wide variety of lean cuts of meats, including pork, lamb, veal, venison and dark chicken meat three to four times a week. Fish may also be eaten.

- Use enriched or fortified cereals if available. Bread and pasta are not fortified in New Zealand. Choose wholegrain breads, pasta, rice and cereals.

- As vitamin C enhances iron absorption serve foods which are rich in this vitamin. Foods high in vitamin C include kiwifruit, oranges, strawberries, rock melon, green peppers, cauliflower and tomato.

- Cooking in cast-iron pots or skillets increases iron content of foods. Curry is high in iron when cooked in this way.

- Tannic acid in tea, phytates in bran and polyphenols in coffee may all reduce or inhibit the absorption of iron. Drink these beverages in moderation and preferably not with meals. Oxylates in vegetables, especially spinach and silverbeet, also inhibit iron absorption.

- Iron in vegetable protein (non-haem iron) is poorly absorbed and should be combined with animal sources (containing haem iron). Forty percent of animal iron is absorbed compared with only 10 percent of plant iron. Some good food combinations are: spinach and liver; spinach and egg; chillibeans and beef; and lentil soup and chicken.

- Some women of reproductive age may require iron supplements. It is recommended that iron medication be taken half an hour before meals (on an empty stomach) with water or fruit juice, but not with milk.

■ *ADEQUATE DAILY INTAKE OF IRON FOR NEW ZEALANDERS*

Infants	6 mg	Women:	12 mg
Children	10 mg	During pregnancy	15 mg
Teenagers	12 mg	During lactation	13 mg
Men	10 mg		

■ ■ ■

Calcium

Calcium is an essential nutrient throughout life for normal body function, teeth and bones. Ninety-nine percent of calcium is located in the bones and teeth. The remaining 1 percent is found in the blood and tissues, especially the muscle. The level of calcium in the blood remains constant and is not affected by the diet. Calcium is the fifth most abundant element in the body and makes up 1.5–2 percent of the total body weight (about 1.2 kg).

Calcium in the bone combines with another mineral, phosphorus, in a ratio of 2:1. Soft drinks that are high in acid and contain large amounts of phosphorus upset this balance. Phosphates also tend to reduce the absorption of iron, calcium and other metals. The teenage sportswoman has a particular need for adequate calcium and increased use of sweet drinks and diet sodas to replace milk is of concern, as this increases the kilojoules and reduces the calcium content of the diet. These women may be placing their future calcium status at risk.

Bone acts as the support structure for the body and a readily available source of calcium for the body's function and metabolism. Calcium plays an important role in blood clotting, muscle contraction, heart muscle function, nerve transmissions, membranes, cell structure and the functioning of various enzymes. Bone is a living tissue and is constantly turning over throughout life. Three to 5 percent of the skeleton is actively remodelled and replaced continuously. The turn-over is higher during periods of growth such as pregnancy, breast-feeding, infancy and the growth spurt of adolescence.

The loss of calcium from bone over a period of time results in actual

101

bone loss or thinning of the bone. The bones become brittle and break or fracture more easily. This is called osteoporosis.

Calcium is deposited in the bones until a person reaches their mid-thirties. After this, calcium is slowly leached from the bone, which becomes thinner and weaker. When the rate of calcium loss from the bone becomes greater than the rate it is deposited, problems arise. This begins around the mid-thirties, but menopause causes this loss to accelerate in women. About 1–1.5 percent of bone mass is lost each year following menopause. A low calcium intake further aggravates bone loss. In men, who have more bone than women (30 percent), bone losses are generally delayed for around seven years compared to women. Often it is too late to repair much of the loss in later years. Encouragement must be given to young sportswomen to obtain a regular and adequate supply of calcium from their teens onwards.

The level of female sex hormones is an important factor. A decrease in oestrogen accelerates bone loss. Other factors that influence bone loss include a high salt diet, a high protein diet, a high intake of alcohol, smoking, a high intake of caffeine and a lack of or excessive exercise.

Stress fractures may occur more often in sportspeople with poor intakes and lowered stores of calcium. Low calcium intake may also be one of the factors involved in high blood pressure (hypertension).

Calcium requirements

What is an adequate daily intake of calcium? Levels have been set for New Zealanders and vary with age, sex, growth phase, diet and metabolism. During periods of growth in childhood, adolescence, during pregnancy and when breastfeeding, calcium requirements are increased.

Age	ADI mg
Infants (0–1 year)	600
Children (1–8 years)	600
Young women (12–17 years)	800
Adult men	600
Adult women*	600
Pregnant women	1 200
Lactating women	1 200

* At present, no level has been set for post-menopausal women but a level of 1 200 mg has been suggested.

■ ■ ■

Foods rich in calcium

Intakes of calcium can easily be obtained by regularly including foods high in this mineral in the diet. By using one of the following menus each day you can maintain a daily calcium intake of 600 mg.

Menu 1 Breakfast	Ca mg
1 cup whole milk	300
30 g cheddar cheese or	
300 g cottage cheese	240
2 slices bread	16
2 fruit (orange and kiwifruit)	62
Total	581

Menu 3 Dessert and snack	Ca mg
½ cup ice cream	165
¼ cup custard	73
½ cup pears	15
4 slices bread	32
40 g cheese	320
Total	605

Menu 4 No dairy products	ca mg
75 g chicken	14
Salad: lettuce	*
¼ cup peanuts	30
1 tbsp almonds	33
1 cup broccoli	136
½ cup carrots	26
½ cup celery	31
½ cup peas	22
½ cup bean salad	83
1 potato	10
½ cup muesli	39
5 dried apricots	23
2 tbsp sesame seeds	38
2 tbsp hazelnut	59
1 orange	37
1 slice fruit cake	40
Total	621

Menu 2 Dinner or lunch	Ca mg
½ tin salmon (180 g)	326
6 mussels	180
1 baked potato	10
1 cup silverbeet	110
Total	626

Menu 5 Vegetarian	Ca mg
½ cup muesli	39
200 g yoghurt	343
2 kiwifruit	25
2 slices bread	16
1 cup baked beans	101
1 baked potato	10
½ cup carrots	26
½ cup cabbage	32
1 pear	15
Total	607

* Contains no measurable calcium.
(Note: Tofu (soya bean curd) is an excellent source of calcium for vegetarians. One cup of tofu equals one cup of milk.) ■ ■ ■

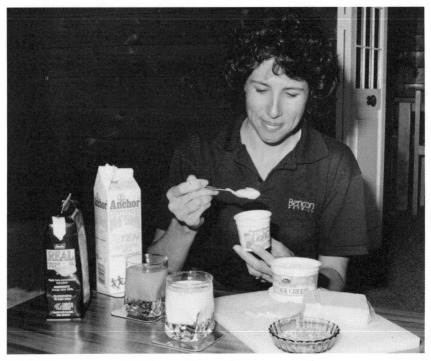

Tracey Fear, New Zealand netball captain in 1988, compares foods for calcium content.

■ SOURCES OF CALCIUM EQUAL TO ONE GLASS OF MILK

The following servings provide approximately 300 mg of calcium:

40 g cheese	1 cup tofu
2 cups cottage cheese	2 cups broccoli
1 cup yoghurt	1½ cups green vegetables
2½ slices processed cheese	16 oysters
75 g camembert cheese	12 large mussels
75 g parmesan cheese	½ cup salmon
40 g gruyere cheese	70 g sardines
1 cup ice cream	100 g shrimps

■ ■ ■

Remember that the calcium found in dairy products is better absorbed than that found in vegetables as the oxalic acid present in vegetables hinders absorption. It is also important to consider the amount of a food eaten. Half a kilogram of broccoli tops contains 600 mg of calcium, but this quantity would be difficult to eat in one sitting.

Excessive calcium and vitamin D

Excessive calcium in the body does not appear to be an advantage. The body is very sensitive to high intakes of some nutrients. Excessive amounts of vitamin D can cause a withdrawal of calcium from the bone and a high level of calcium in the blood. These high blood levels are often associated with kidney stones, muscle and bone changes and, in some animals, bleeding from the gut. The key to calcium is to have a balanced diet made up of a wide variety of foods, including some rich sources on a regular basis. The athlete should pay attention to maintaining adequate levels of dietary calcium, but avoid excesses.

Summary

Training meals for any sportsperson should provide 55–60 percent of energy from carbohydrates (increased to 70 percent for hard training), 15 percent protein and the remainder should be supplied by fat. A protein intake around 1.5 g per kilogram per day is suitable for most athletes, with an increase to 2 g for some. Excessive protein has no advantage. The disadvantages include a reduction in the proportion of carbohydrate and an increase in saturated fats. In addition, the excess nitrogen must be excreted and this excretion process requires additional water.

If the bulk of complex carbohydrates is uncomfortable for some individuals, simple carbohydrates may be increased to provide sufficient energy. Frequent small meals may be more suitable. The inclusion of fresh fruits and vegetables will provide adequate intakes of vitamins and minerals. Iron levels may require assessment in susceptible individuals and calcium intakes require monitoring in women performing endurance activities. Sufficient fluid is essential to avoid dehydration. Athletes must consume fluids to replace losses and this replacement may take several hours. Remember that thirst is not an adequate indicator of hydration.

There is no magic diet that will enhance performance, but practising with different eating patterns and selecting foods appropriate to the demands of training and competition will enable athletes to compete at levels of maximum performance. An inadequate, incomplete or unbalanced diet will undo much of the effort put into training.

13 Energy

For the human body to function it needs energy. Energy is essential for breathing, growth, movement and exercise, and to enable the heart to beat. The muscle is provided with energy for activity in the form of a substance called *adenosine triphosphate* (ATP). ATP is the product resulting from the breakdown of glucose and is the basic unit of energy for muscle contraction, such as for one lift of a weight, one push, or one sit-up. The body has a limited supply of ATP stored in the muscle; body reserves are depleted in 1–2 seconds.

The energy for any further muscle contraction in the body is provided by three energy systems: the phosphocreatine system (the small body-stores), which provides instant energy; the short circuit energy system forming lactic acid (anaerobic glycolysis); and the extended glycogen or aerobic system.

The phosphocreatine system

No oxygen is required for this system, which means it is anaerobic (producing energy independent of oxygen). Instant energy for sudden movement and a few repetitions of weightlifting are supplied by this system. The energy is provided by high energy phosphate substances in the muscle and lasts for 5–10 seconds. Eighty-five grams of ATP are stored in the body at one time. Therefore, ATP must be resynthesised to provide a continuous supply of energy. Although this energy is readily used it is also rapidly replaced; 50 percent is available in 30 seconds and 100 percent in 2 minutes. Weightlifting is an example of a dynamic burst of energy using this system.

The lactic acid system

If exercise continues the muscle must rely on carbohydrates to manufacture ATP. In the absence of oxygen (anaerobic) stored carbohydrate can be broken down to supply energy for the muscle contraction. Carbohydrate is provided by stored glycogen, blood glucose and liver glycogen.

The carbohydrate, as glycogen, is converted into glucose and travels via the bloodstream to the muscle. Lactic acid is then produced. If intense activity is maintained lactic acid accumulates in the muscle and blood causing fatigue. It may be 45-60 minutes before it is removed from the system. The lactic acid system provides a rapid supply of ATP for intense short bursts of energy. It can also be an energy reserve for the final sprint (exhaustion occurs in approximately 60-90 seconds). Tolerance to lactic acid varies with training and fitness. Resting between a series of repetitions appears to enhance gains in muscle tone and strength.

The aerobic system

For long periods of training the body switches to the aerobic system, which requires oxygen. The aerobic system is the breakdown of stored carbohydrate and fat in the presence of oxygen to supply energy for muscle contraction. Carbohydrate is supplied from the glycogen in muscle, circulating blood glucose and liver glycogen, and fat is provided from fat stores (adipose tissue). This energy system supplies the fuel for endurance events.

Sportspeople have the ability to use one or any combination of these systems. Different sports demand different types and amounts of muscular activity. Therefore, different muscle fibres and energy systems are required for different sports. The sprinter depends on the anaerobic energy system and the marathon runner uses the aerobic energy system. In games and team events a combination of all systems is used.

Energy for exercise is provided through the food you eat. If you eat more than you use for energy the excess is stored as fat. The process of converting food inside the body into energy is called metabolism. The speed at which this happens is called the metabolic rate.

Fuels for energy

A **kilocalorie**, usually referred to simply as a Calorie, is a unit of heat used to express the energy value of a food. One Cal is the amount of heat needed to increase the temperature of 1 kg of water by 1 degree celsius. One Cal equals 4.2 kilojoules (kJ). The energy value of a food can be measured directly by the amount of heat given off when the food is burned. Specialised equipment is required to perform this measurement.

A 68 kg athlete has around 166 200 Cal of energy stored in the body. Of this, 1 200 Cal are from carbohydrate, 25 000 from protein. The largest contributor is fat, with the potential to supply 140 000 Cal of energy.

■ ENERGY VALUES

1 g fat provides 9 Cal (38 kJ)*
1 g alcohol provides 7 Cal (30 kJ)
1 g protein provides 4 Cal (17 kJ)
1 g carbohydrate provides 4 Cal (17 kJ)

* 1 Cal equals 4.2 kJ (kilojoules), 1000 kJ = 1 MJ (megajoule).

It is easy to see that fat provides the most energy per gram or unit of food. However, fat is slowly digested; digestion can take up to 4 hours, whereas protein requires around 3 hours, and carbohydrate clears the stomach within 2 hours. Fat is also associated with a number of health problems.

Optimum energy intake

The following recommendations are suggested as the most suitable proportions of total food intake to promote the best possible performance.

Beginning with the proportions illustrated in stage one in the following table, the athlete can adapt to many of the recommended changes in the baseline. For training, further refinement is possible by moving on to stage two. Sportsmen and sportswomen may find the change from the typical New Zealand diet to stage two an extreme change and compliance may be difficult.

	Stage 1	Stage 2
Carbohydrate	55%	60-65%
Protein	15-20%	15-20%
Fat	25-30%	20-25%

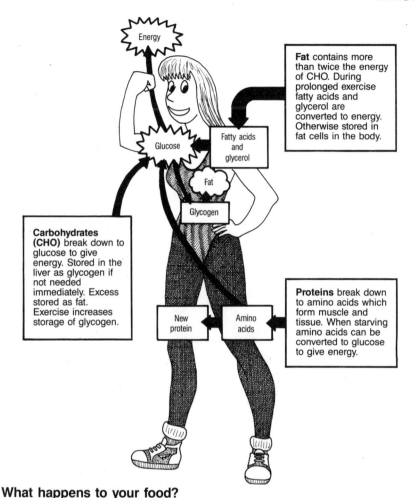

Energy

Fat contains more than twice the energy of CHO. During prolonged exercise fatty acids and glycerol are converted to energy. Otherwise stored in fat cells in the body.

Glucose

Fatty acids and glycerol

Fat

Glycogen

Carbohydrates (CHO) break down to glucose to give energy. Stored in the liver as glycogen if not needed immediately. Excess stored as fat. Exercise increases storage of glycogen.

New protein

Amino acids

Proteins break down to amino acids which form muscle and tissue. When starving amino acids can be converted to glucose to give energy.

What happens to your food?

In some cases it may be necessary to alter these basic levels. Carbohydrate can be increased and the fat content lowered for some endurance events. These proportions indicate a food pattern that is high in carbohydrate, with a moderate level of protein and fat. The high carbohydrate foods should be of the complex type. This includes cereals, pasta, rice, bread, potatoes, fruit and vegetables.

Glucose and glycogen

Glucose is the most common and one of the smallest carbohydrate units (others include fructose and galactose). Glucose performs three roles in energy release:

■ ENERGY CONTENT OF SOME FOODS

Food	Serving	Energy kJ
Pizza	1	1152
Scone	1	461
Spaghetti	1	419
Meat and spaghetti	1	1466
Fried flounder	1	754
Fish in sauce	2	1466
Battered fish	1	1676
Cornflakes	1 cup	445
Muesli	1 cup	1978
Weetbix	2	420
Iced sponge	1 slice	1613
Doughnut	1	1550

■ ■ ■

- It is used directly for energy.

- It replenishes glycogen stores.

- Surplus to body needs is converted to fat.

The role of glycogen can be compared in general terms to the role of starch in plants. Animal tissues contain no starch molecules so must use glycogen to perform a similar function. Glycogen is not present in any significant amount in food. Carbohydrate foods are digested and the resulting glucose enters the liver and muscle; if this glucose is not used immediately for energy it is stored as glycogen. This process is called glycogenesis. Under normal circumstances, the body has the capacity to store around 400 g of glycogen. This glycogen can be transferred back into glucose in the liver to provide energy when required by the exercising muscle (glycolysis). Carbohydrate loading elevates these levels.

When glycogen stores are depleted, as with repeated bursts of intense activity or endurance events, the body must use other fuel sources. Protein and fats are then used to provide glucose for muscle activity. Even though fat is an energy source it is not as readily available and is less efficient than glycogen stores.

Carbohydrate

Individuals actively involved in sports activities should depend on carbohydrate for their energy requirements.

Carbohydrate should provide the majority of an active individual's energy needs. During training this should be a minimum of 50–55 percent. Some competitive events or long endurance training may require an increase to 60–80 percent. To allow for this increase in carbohydrate consumption a decrease in fat content is necessary.

Factors which affect energy requirements

To estimate the daily energy requirements of an individual the following factors must be taken into account.

● The metabolic rate — basal metabolism (energy needed at rest)

● Energy expenditure of physical activity or exercise

● Specific dynamic action of food.

Basal metabolic rate (BMR)

This is the amount of energy (expressed in Calories or kilojoules) needed to maintain:

● Regulation of body temperature

● Cell activity

● Respiration (breathing)

● Heart-beat and circulation.

Establishing the BMR provides a baseline for estimating the number of kilojoules or Calories required for energy and activity. Several methods are available to estimate BMR; for example, nomographs show height and weight relative to surface area.

The following factors have an effect on the BMR:

Body composition Females have a 5–10 percent lower BMR than males because they carry more fat and less lean tissue. Athletes have a higher percentage of lean body mass and a 5 percent higher BMR than non-athletic individuals.

Age BMR is highest during periods of rapid growth; children have higher metabolic rates than adolescents or adults. The BMR declines around 2 percent per decade or 15 percent from 20 to 60 years (see graph below). To maintain weight in the later years of life, exercise must play a more important role.

Sex   Males have a higher BMR than females. This helps to explain why males reduce weight at a faster rate than females.

Physical health   The metabolic rate can decrease as much as 50 percent with starvation, disease or while following extremely low energy diets. Lean muscle tissue is lost, adaptive mechanisms take over and the body conserves energy.

Pregnancy   An increase of almost 28 percent in BMR has been reported in pregnant women compared to the non-pregnant. This is due to the development of the reproductive organs and the foetus. Increases are also seen in respiration and cardiac output, or heart rate.

Climate   Individuals who live in tropical climates appear to have a lower BMR compared to those living in cold or temperate climates. As the climate for most people is relatively constant the overall effect on BMR is minimal.

Physical activity

The most significant influence on energy expenditure is regular (daily) physical activity. Exercise can increase the metabolic rate for over 24 hours after the activity. The following illustrations show some examples of the energy cost of various activities (to convert to kilojoules multiply Calories by 4.2):

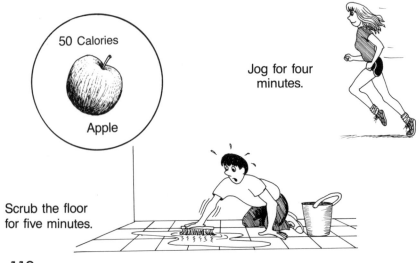

50 Calories

Apple

Jog for four minutes.

Scrub the floor for five minutes.

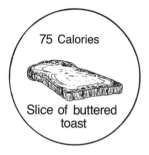

75 Calories

Slice of buttered toast

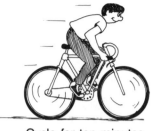

Cycle for ten minutes.

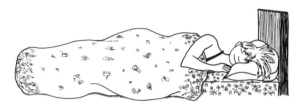

Sleep for one and a half hours.

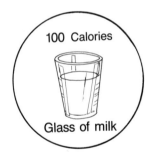

100 Calories

Glass of milk

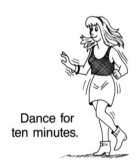

Dance for ten minutes.

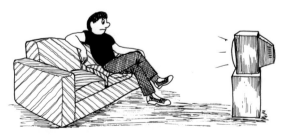

Watch TV for one and a quarter hours.

113

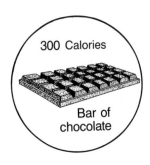

300 Calories

Bar of chocolate

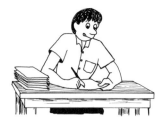

Sit a three hour exam.

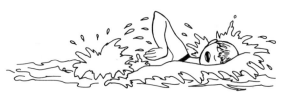

Swim round a pool for 45 minutes without touching the sides.

Remember that body size influences the energy cost of exercise. A heavy person expends more energy than a light person in weight-bearing exercises such as jogging and walking because a greater mass is moved.

Specific dynamic action of foods

The specific dynamic action of food refers to the amount of heat generated by eating and digesting food. It makes only a minimal contribution to energy requirements.

After oxygen and water, food is the third most important element for life. It is the crucial element for the athlete and sportsperson to provide fuel for activity. The number of kilojoules or Calories needed varies, depending on body size, age, activity level and BMR. It is difficult to determine individual needs accurately. Adequate energy content and a balance of all other nutrients (carbohydrate, protein, fat, vitamins, minerals and water) will provide optimum nutritional status.

Adequate energy allows the sportsperson to maintain ideal or desirable body weight range and is easily provided through the consumption of a wide variety of foods. It is important that people actively involved in sports activity consider the source of energy in the food plan. Remember, no single food provides all the nutrients in the correct amount or proportion essential to maintain and promote good health and performance.

■ FOOD INTAKE COMPARED WITH ENERGY EXPENDITURE

The following table shows the number of kilojoules expended per minute for a variety of activities.

	Walk	Cycle	Box	Swim	Squash	Run
Kilojoules expended per minute	22	34	41	47	63	82

On this basis, it is possible to calculate the length of time spent on each activity to use up the energy contained in specific foods.

Energy intake			Activity in minutes					
Food	Serving	kJ	Walk	Cycle	Box	Swim	Squash	Run
Apple	1	251	12	7	6	5	4	3
Banana	1	398	18	12	10	8	6	4
Kiwifruit	1	126	6	4	3	2.5	2	1.5
Carrot	1 cup	188	9	6	5	4	3	2
Corn cob	1 med	587	27	17	14	12	9	7
Kumara	½ cup	419	19	12	10	9	6.5	5
Soya beans	½ cup	503	23	15	12	11	8	6
Kidney beans	½ cup	472	21	14	11.5	10	7.5	6
Chow mein	1	817	37	24	20	17	13	10
Fried chicken	1	1227	56	36	30	26	19	15
Hamburger	1	1781	81	52	43	38	28	22
Paté	¼ cup	1047	48	31	25.5	22	16.5	13
Beer (glass)	1	440	20	13	11	9	7	5
Wine (white)	1	377	17	11	9	8	6	4.5
Cheese slices	2 (50 g)	922	42	27	22.5	19.5	14.5	11
Choco ice cream	1	628	28	18.5	15	13	10	7.5
Milkshake	1	1466	67	43	36	31	23	18
Lemon & Paeroa	1	419	19	12	10	9	6.5	5
Cola soda	1	400	18	12	10	8.5	6	5
Moro bar	1	1244	56	36.5	30	26.5	20	15

Values for a 68 kg male. To convert to calories divide kJ per activity by 4.2. For example, 1 banana equals 95 Calories (398÷4.2), 5.2 Calories/minute walking.

■ ■ ■

14
Weight gain

There are times when it is desirable to gain weight to improve performance in a particular sport. Shot putters, hammer and discus throwers, heavyweight wrestlers, rugby and rugby league front row players all require maximum muscle mass for strength and bulk.

Increased weight should be seen as an increase in muscle weight, not just body weight. If the weight increase is an increase in fat the expected benefits and improvements in performance will not occur. The increase in fat tissue exposes sportspeople to a number of health problems, apart from obesity.

Gaining muscle mass or lean body weight requires a different technique to losing body-fat weight. An increase in energy intake is necessary, but the quality of this food is just as important. The increased food intake should provide a balance of all nutrients, not just the high energy foods such as sugar, pies and desserts. Any increase in muscle mass also requires resistance exercise, such as weight training. Without the increase in exercise the additional food eaten will be converted into fat stores.

Guidelines

The following points should be considered when following a weight gain programme:

- Increase intake by 500 Cal (2.1 MJ) per day.
- Include moderate exercise.

- Aim for a gradual increase in weight.
- Eat regular-sized meals and snacks.
- Watch the intake of fatty and salty foods.
- Do not use artificial or chemical means to gain weight.
- Increase the energy intake earlier in the day.

The requirements of the sport and the health and physique of the individual sportsperson must also be considered. Each sport has a unique set of demands which are a characteristic part of the sport. It is necessary for some sportspeople to gain weight and muscle size to provide an advantage in strength and performance, but there are other sports in which an increase in muscle would be a disadvantage, for example triathlons, ballet and sports which require a great deal of flexibility.

It is important that before a weight gain programme is embarked on the family history of the sportsperson is checked for evidence of heart disease, high blood pressure and diabetes. Remember that an increase in weight occurs with age in many people. By assessing the family background it is possible to see if a sportsperson has inherited a trim body type.

Increased food intake

To gain weight it is necessary to consume around 2.1 MJ per day in addition to the normal food eaten. The easiest way to add this amount of energy is to include snacks during the day. Below is a list of foods that provide this amount of energy as a snack.

> 5–6 glasses orange juice
> 2 peanut butter sandwiches (4 slices bread)
> 5 pieces fresh fruit (bananas or apples)
> 2½ cups fresh fruit salad
> 2 average slices pizza
> 4 medium potatoes
> 2 milkshakes
> 1 large cup dried fruit
> 90 g various nuts
> 80 g cheese and 5 crackers
> 2 cups fruit-flavoured yoghurt (low fat)
> 2 muesli bars (plain)

One pound or 0.5 kg of lean muscle tissue equals 10.5 MJ and

117

the same weight of fat contains 14.7 MJ. Lean tissue contains more water, protein and carbohydrate than fat and therefore weighs more. One kg of fat takes up 20 percent more room than 1 kg of muscle.

Increased exercise

An increase in energy input must be accompanied by an increase in exercise, especially resistance exercise such as weight training. This promotes muscle growth rather than depositing fat. If you stop exercising, muscle will not turn into fat as muscle cells are incapable of turning into fat cells. What occurs with inactivity is a change in the distribution of muscle mass and fat weight. As fat deposits decline with activity the muscle contours become more visible. With inactivity the muscles shrink, and as less energy is burned fat deposits increase, creating the illusion that muscle turns into fat.

Gradual weight increase

There is a limit to how fast lean weight gain can be achieved. Aim for 500 g a week and check body fat percentage regularly.

Regular-sized meals

Eat regularly and avoid consuming large meals. Do not try to force feed. Stop when you feel full. Increase the energy content by adding more snacks or eating six medium-sized meals a day. Balance the consumption of food with the expenditure of energy throughout the day. This promotes a healthier eating pattern. Once weight gain has been achieved to the desired level, maintaining the weight involves a slight modification of the eating patterns and reducing snacks, rather than a total change in eating.

Care with fat and salt

When selecting foods, remember that fats are the most concentrated source of energy. Generally, New Zealanders consume more than adequate fat in their diet, so it is not desirable to encourage any further intake. Protein foods tend to have a fat component and large intakes of protein are not recommended. To improve energy intake and provide fuel for additional exercise, increase the energy from a carbohydrate source.

Foods for weight increase

Here are some tips to increase weight through good quality food choices.

Fruit   Add lightly stewed fruit to cereals, in lunches, with ice cream or as snacks. Take care to choose canned fruit in light syrup only or cooked in its own juice. Dried fruit such as bananas, pineapples, pears, raisins, dates and apricots contain more energy than the fresh variety. Fresh fruits with higher energy values include bananas, berry fruits, mangoes, pawpaws and pineapples.

Fruit juices   These fluids are easily added to the food plan without increasing the bulk. Apple, orange, pineapple, apricot and blackberry juices contain more kilojoules than tomato and grapefruit. To increase the energy value use one-third less water than recommended for concentrates.

Milk and dairy products   The addition of skim milk powder to milk drinks (glasses of milk, milkshakes, yoghurt shakes) and custard increases the energy content of the beverage. High energy flavours such as Milo, drinking chocolate, Nestle's Quik or other milkshake flavourings can also be added. If these drinks are made in bulk and consumed during the day, store under refrigeration. Any remaining after 24 hours should be discarded. These drinks make excellent ice blocks if frozen (double the flavouring). Selecting low fat dairy products (milk, cheese and yoghurt) keeps the saturated fat content at a lower level.

Bread and cereals   Use generous amounts of peanut butter and spreads on bread and toast. Use thick toast-sliced bread to make Dagwood sandwiches. Choose bread that is heavier per slice, rather than slim or light sliced bread. Wholegrain bread or sports breads tend to be denser and thicker, containing more energy. Cook hot cereals such as porridge or muesli porridge with milk instead of water. This increases the energy content and the nutritional value of the cereal. Skim milk or fruit-flavoured yoghurt can be added to the cereal, or porridge can be cooked with dried apricots or raisins or topped with fresh fruit, such as apple, banana or apricots. Breakfast cereals can be eaten as desserts or snacks during the day. Add fruit, yoghurt or raisins as toppings in addition to milk. Muesli and heavier cereals contain higher energy values per serving than rice bubbles and cornflakes. Add extra dried fruit and more nuts to muesli.

Meats   It is not necessary to dramatically increase the serving sizes of meat portions as this may increase the intake of saturated fat; this applies to lamb, beef, pork and veal. Eat these foods in moderation. Chicken and fish have lower energy levels and lower saturated fat contents. Increase the energy content of these meats by crumbing and coating (use cornflakes, wholegrain bread crumbs,

119

bran or malt biscuit crumbs and seasoned flour) and lightly cook in oil. The addition of sauces such as white sauce, cheese sauce or wine increases the energy value.

Vegetables Vegetables can generally be divided into two groups, one of which contains a higher kilojoule content. This group includes peas, potatoes, kumara, yams, corn, beetroot, broad beans, parsnip, squash and taro. Topping vegetables with grated cheese, cheese sauce, flavoured white sauce or sautéd bread crumbs, or adding sour cream, gravy, margarine or almond slivers will increase the energy content. Many of these vegetables are excellent as fritters. Skim milk powder, margarine or an egg can be added to mashed vegetables such as potato, carrots and parsnip or pumpkin. The lower energy vegetables can be stuffed with rice, legumes or nuts to increase energy content.

Salads These are generally considered low energy meals, but carbohydrate, protein and energy are easily increased with the addition of cottage cheese, dry roasted peanuts, sunflower seeds, pumpkin seeds, croutons (baked, not fried), chopped nuts (walnuts, hazelnuts, peanuts), salmon and tuna, chunks of fresh fruit (apple, orange, peach, nectarine or mango), and small amounts of grilled bacon and lean meat. Use generous servings of fat-reduced dressings to keep the saturated fat level down.

Legumes, nuts and seeds These foods can be added to salads, casseroles, soups and vegetable dishes. Used as toppings, they provide variety as well as increased energy content. Beans are an excellent source of protein and carbohydrate. Examples include soya, kidney and lima beans; split peas; and haricot and baked beans.

Desserts Adding cereals such as rice bubbles, cornflakes or muesli to fruit and custard makes a tempting treat or dessert. Consider other alternatives to standard puddings — for example, fruit-flavoured muffins, fruit cake, fruit biscuits, crumbed fruit fritters and fruit kebabs. Try rice pudding with raisins or other dried fruit, ice cream with crushed biscuits and nuts, carrot cake and custard, or banana muffins with vanilla sauce.

Soups Garnishing soups with croutons, cheese (parmesan or low fat varieties such as gouda, edam, brie, camembert), or a kob of margarine, are simple ways to add kilojoules. If using canned soup add milk, evaporated milk or skim milk in place of water. To packet soups or one-cup soups add rice, noodles or beans. Lentils, corn, split peas, barley, noodles, rice and beans can all be added to home-made or canned soups.

Snacks Choosing more substantial snacks that provide a higher intake of all nutrients may be sufficient in itself to produce weight gain in some sportspeople. Selecting snacks of a high nutritional quality provides a healthier intake. A snack in the evening may be suitable for some, but others may prefer to consume smaller snacks during the day. Healthy snacks include dried fruit, nuts, bran muffins, wholemeal scones, pizza, milkshakes, banana, chocolate milk drinks, sandwiches, sunflower seeds, pumpkin seeds, fruit shakes, cheese and crackers.

Alcohol Drinking a glass of wine, sherry, beer or spirit before a meal can stimulate the appetite. However, it is important to keep intakes to a moderate level. Alcohol provides little nutrient benefit except for energy, and excessive intakes replace meals. Because of the dehydrating effect of alcohol, the intake of other fluids, such as water, juice or milk, must be maintained.

Menus for weight gain, loss and maintenance

Three members of a college rugby team have different targets to meet regarding their respective weights. Peter needs to decrease his weight by 4 kg, Jason's weight is fine and Greg needs to increase his weight by 5 kg. Compare the changes made to the baseline eating patterns of these three individuals to achieve their desired results.

■ *MENUS*

Jason — to maintain weight	Peter — to decrease weight		Greg — to increase weight	
		SAVE kJ		ADD kJ
Breakfast	**Breakfast**		**Breakfast**	
1 cup orange juice				
1 cup toasted muesli				
1 cup 2% milk	Use trim milk	— 100		
2 slices wholemeal bread				
2 tsp raspberry jam	Only 1 tsp jam	— 135		
2 tsp butter	Only 1 tsp butter	— 190		
1 fruit				

121

Lunch	Lunch	Lunch	
75 g lean meat (pork) 25 g cheese (1 slice) 2 tsp butter 2 slices wholemeal bread salad filling 1 fruit 1 fruit yoghurt	Only 1 tsp butter Add 1 fruit + 222 Move yoghurt to - 848 dinner	1 tsp butter 2 slices wholemeal	+ 190 + 482
1 banana sandwich (2 slices bread) 1 tsp butter	Fruit only Remove bread - 480 Delete butter - 190	Fruit juice 1 cup 1 tsp butter	+ 460 + 190

Dinner	Dinner	Dinner	
100 g chicken 2 baked potatoes 1 cup peas 1 cup carrots ½ cup fresh fruit salad ½ cup plain ice cream	Remove ice cream - 1 050 Replace with yoghurt + 848	1 tsp sour cream + 152 ½ cup fruit salad + 200 1 cup 2% milk + 472	
Total change	- 2113		+ 2146

Nutrient analysis

Jason			*Peter*			*Greg*		
Energy	12 MJ (2 800 Cal)		Energy	9.8 MJ (2 300 Cal)		Energy	14 MJ (3 300 Cal)	
CHO	60%	419 g	CHO	66%	380 g	CHO	59%	491 g
Fat	24%	79 g	Fat	16%	43 g	Fat	25%	93 g
Protein	16%	119 g	Protein	18%	108 g	Protein	16%	138 g

■ ■ ■

15
Weight loss

Reducing weight and attempting to change body shape has become a popular pursuit for many people, but few actually achieve long-term success. In Auckland, a study investigating the prevalence of obesity showed that 48 percent of the men from 35 to 64 years were overweight (8 percent were obese) and 38 percent of the women were overweight (10 percent obese). Overweight or obese individuals have an increased incidence of high blood pressure, coronary heart disease, diabetes and raised blood fats.

Often, attempts to reduce body fat or weight become a continuous campaign, retreating with success then counter-attacking if the weight is regained. This yoyo or rollercoaster approach to weight loss must be avoided. Many weight-conscious people assume a reduction in weight is the result of a loss of fat, or that a weight gain is an increase in body fat levels.

There are some sports in which weight loss may be required to allow an individual to compete in a particular event or class. Sports participants who need to be concerned about weight include gymnasts, figure skaters, jockeys, wrestlers, bodybuilders, boxers and rowers. Some runners mistakenly believe the lighter they are, the faster they will run. There is no evidence to support this.

Once the sportsperson has assessed his or her body mass index (BMI), body fat percentages are determined, the decision to reduce weight made, and a sensible programme can be developed. It is important that the energy level provided by carbohydrate in the food plan is not unnecessarily restricted. Anyone engaged in serious physical exercise must realise the importance of this nutrient in providing energy for training and sports performance. Weight loss should be achieved before competition. Sportspeople cannot compete or perform effectively while on weight loss programmes. For each individual there is an optimum body weight at which physical efficiency peaks. Other factors to be considered are age, body surface area, growth, exercise levels, present body composition and long-term goals. The optimum or desirable body weight is not a set figure but more a range that varies with each individual and within each of the different sports. Weight measured on scales does not evaluate body composition and only measures the change in weight, not the actual quality of the weight lost. Weight loss can be caused by dehydration, muscle metabolism or loss in fat tissue.

Dieting itself may cause weight gain. As the sportsperson attempts to reduce weight by using many new 'improved', modified or updated diets, changes in metabolism can occur. Any organism repeatedly deprived of food, such as occurs with continuous restrictive dieting, increases the chances of survival by learning to store food more efficiently. Reacting to a diet is like reacting to a famine. The body may reduce basal metabolism to obtain more mileage out of less fuel. This may explain why some people find weight reduction difficult.

After exercise, the metabolic rate of the body remains raised for several hours and further energy is burned in addition to that used for exercise. More fat and less muscle mass is lost when dieters increase their activity and raise their energy expenditure. However, the type of exercise performed does make a difference. As fat is not used for fuel until 20–30 minutes of activity has passed, exercising at moderate levels for long periods of time is more effective for weight loss than short bursts of strenuous exercise.

Factors that influence weight loss

Timing
Is this the right time to concentrate on weight loss? Has sufficient time been allocated to losing weight steadily and slowly? Is the timetable realistic? Many people attempting to reduce weight set themselves unrealistic weight loss timetables, or programmes are started during periods of stress or instability. Take all social factors, such as lifestyle, training and living environment, into consideration.

Motivation
Does the weight reducer have the right mental attitude? Can the benefits of reducing excess body fat be easily explained, identified

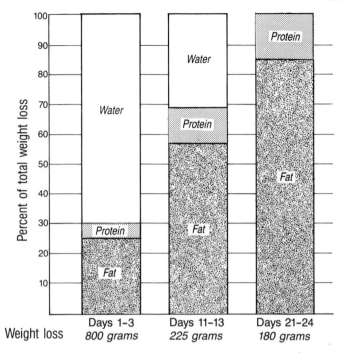

Analysis of weight loss during 24-day weight loss programme involving forced exercise.

(Adapted from Grande, F. Nutrition and energy balance in body composition studies. In *Techniques for Measuring Body Composition*). National Academy of Sciences — National Research Council, Washington, D.C., 1961.)

and understood in terms of enhanced sports performance and improved overall general health?

Choosing the correct diet

Carefully select a programme that brings about weight loss from the fat stores *gradually*. There is no room for fad diets or quick weight loss programmes that will cause sports performance to suffer. The energy requirement provided in the food plan should be obtained from a wide variety of food and be balanced in terms of nutrients. A reduction of 2 100 kJ (500 Cal) a day is a reduction of 14.7 MJ (3 500 Cal) per week, or 500 g (1 lb) of excess body fat. Weight loss programmes that promise a magic ingredient, special forumula or fast weight loss are not appropriate for sportspeople — or anyone, for that matter. Many of these fad diets lead to dehydration and loss of muscle tissue. Weight loss should be within the region of 0.5-1 kg per week (1-2 lb). This slower weight loss causes less mental stress and reduces the effects of fatigue.

125

Changes in eating behaviour

Once the excess weight is lost, the eating patterns that lead to this loss should become part of the permanent changes in eating hehaviour to maintain weight loss. Following eating patterns that lead to boredom, uninteresting meals and inflexible food choices will not provide the encouragement or motivation necessary to maintain the desirable weight once it is reached. Very restrictive dieting leads to bingeing and guilt-eating behaviour. It is far better to take a few weeks longer and make behaviour changes a permanent part of your eating patterns. Aim for success, not perfection.

Water

Water consumption does not cause weight gain in sportspeople and is important for all body functions. Water helps to dilute the by-products of metabolism excreted by the kidneys and avoids dehydration.

Exercise

Body fat should be reduced through the combination of modifying energy input (dieting) and increasing energy expenditure (exercise). This helps to ensure that body fat stores, rather than lean muscle tissue, are reduced.

Steps to reduce body weight

Step 1   Decide on a realistic goal. Set short-term and long-term goals. Identify rewards and benefits to sports performance, such as faster times, improved endurance and health.

Step 2   Determine a rational weight loss timetable. Weight should be checked once or twice a week at the same time wearing the same clothes if possible. Plot results on a graph. Remember that a few days before a sportswoman commences menstruation her weight may increase. Skinfold and body measurements should also be checked at regular intervals.

Step 3   Keep a food diary. This will identify any areas of imbalance in nutritional intake and also show up areas for improvement; for example, skipped or missed meals occurring at a particular time of the week or problems with eating behaviour at certain times of the day, such as in the afternoon or around supper time. Activity levels should also be recorded. It is often useful to mark the consumption of glasses of water and other beverages to estimate intakes.

Step 4 Monitor the energy levels of the eating programme carefully. Never allow the energy level to drop too low. This is why individual programmes are essential. Very low calorie intake drastically impedes sports performance because weight loss results from losses in muscle tissue and dehydration, and fatigue, dizziness and loss of concentration occur. Any weight loss programme that involves a daily consumption of less than 4.2 kilojoules will require vitamin or mineral supplementation and is not recommended for anyone actively involved in sport.

Step 5 Sportspeople should follow an eating pattern based on the nutritional guidelines outlined throughout this book. By increasing the bulk (fibre, salads and vegetables) hunger is delayed. Drinking hot beverages during the winter warms the body and reduces the effects of hunger.

Step 6 Encourage regular meals and distribute food intake throughout the day. Some sportspeople prefer to eat three meals a day while others like to spread the total amount of food over five or six smaller meals. Smaller meals more often satisfy appetite, but care is needed with snacks. Snacks should be of a high nutritional quality and not high in sugar, salt or fat. Missing meals reduces a sportsperson's energy intakes and hence the effectiveness and benefit of training. Foods missed earlier in the day may lead to overcompensation at the following meals.

Step 7 Water is an important nutrient and should be consumed regularly, even when not thirsty. Water is the preferred fluid but small amounts of diet soda and cordials may be used.

Step 8 Behaviour modification strategies help maintain motivation and discipline. Highlight the benefits to be gained from weight loss. Set a reward for achieving both the short-term and long-term goals. Reinforce positive changes in eating and initiative. To maintain weight loss programmes, the sportsperson should learn to manipulate eating patterns to cope with changes in lifestyle and training schedules.

Step 9 Assess progress on the weight loss programme. As the long-term goal draws nearer the amount of weight lost slows down. Check that muscular strength is not deteriorating and speed is maintained. Watch for signs of early fatigue, inattentiveness and unexplained changes in personality. Bodybuilders undergo dramatic changes in temperament close to competition because of the drastic losses in body weight and body fat associated with the coming-down phase. Rapid losses in weight may induce similar effects.

Step 10 Maintain a realistic weight loss once achieved. Avoid wide swings from weight loss to weight gain. It is more realistic to set the desirable weight a little higher, where it is easily maintained, than to have to struggle to maintain a lower weight. Unrealistic weight loss goals could tempt the athlete or sportsperson to resort to undesirable methods, such as using laxatives, vomiting or taking diuretics. If forced to crash diet, carbohydrate stored in muscle will be depleted in 24–48 hours of semi-starvation. The chemical and water balance of the body is disrupted and this may influence hydration. These factors all limit sports performance. Aim to maintain weight during the off-season as well as through the season and life-long, sound nutritional habits will be developed.

Suitable replacement foods

The most effective way to reduce weight is to make small changes in the type and quality of food taken into the body. Gradually these changes will become part of your permanent eating behaviour, rather than a separate set of eating patterns used just to reduce weight.

Fruit Use the natural sweetness found in fruit rather than adding sugar. Take a slightly smaller serving if bottled or canned fruit has been preserved with sugar. Select fruit preserved in its own juice, light syrup or 'no sugar added' syrups. By using fresh fruit with a firmer texture rather than the processed version a feeling of fullness will occur; for example, use fresh apple sliced onto cereal instead of apple sauce. More chewing is involved and the fibre content is higher. Choose the lower energy fruits such as watermelon, honeydew melon, rhubarb, apricots, berry fruit, persimmons, tamarillo, pepino, and red and black currants.

Fruit juices By drinking a glass of fruit juice a day over 650 kJ can be added. This is equal to three oranges. It is much easier to drink the juice and remain hungry, but three oranges will provide sufficient fibre to create a feeling of fullness. Dilute fruit juice at least 50/50 with water. Many fruit juices today are marketed on the concept that no sugar is added, but some are more concentrated. The sugar naturally present in the fruit acts as a preservative. One glass of fruit juice can contain over three teaspoons of sugar. Tomato juices are lower in energy value, but care is needed because of the sodium content.

Milk By changing from the traditional dairy products to skim and trim milk, low fat yoghurts, and low fat cheeses, the amount of fat normally found in this food group is reduced. Cheddar cheese is over one-third fat (35 percent). Selecting a lower fat cheese such as cottage (3 percent), mozzarella (18 percent), or brie and camembert (23 percent fat) can reduce the fat content of a meal yet will still provide adequate calcium.

Bread and cereals Use the wholegrain variety and a minimal amount of butter or margarine. Use peanut butter or butter, not both. Go easy on spreads such as jam, honey and marmalade. Remove as much added sugar as possible. Use thin bread rather than thick toast slices. It is not necessary to remove bread and cereals from the food plan when reducing weight. Crackers, preferably wholemeal, are generally low in energy content, but read the label as many have high saturated fat contents. Select foods which provide energy from carbohydrate sources and supply a wide range of other nutrients such as vitamins and minerals. Try not to snack between meals. Limit biscuits, cake, sweets and other snack food. This includes muesli bars which can be high in sugar and fat.

Meats Eating smaller slices of lean meat will provide adequate protein, iron and zinc for sportspeople. Remove all the fat (including the skin on chicken) before and after cooking. Eat kebabs, stir fry, Chinese, and other dishes that require small amounts of meat rather than large servings of steaks and chops. When comparing one 200 g steak to five baked potatoes, each potato filled with two teaspoons of sour cream, it is surprising to learn they contain an equal amount of energy. Yet how often do you see dieters skip the potato and eat the steak? Meats contain hidden fat which must be accounted for when reducing weight. Steam, bake, grill and microwave rather than fry or roast. Swap the gravy or white sauce for another serving of vegetables.

Vegetables Include a wide range of vegetables in the meals. At least four servings per day from the fruit and vegetable group are recommended. If you are hungry, include more vegetables that are lower in energy value but try not to add toppings such as grated cheese, white sauces, butter, margarine, dressing and sour cream.

129

When mashing potatoes use trim milk only. The method of cooking food can make a considerable difference to its energy content.

■ *ENERGY CONTENT OF 100 G POTATO USING DIFFERENT COOKING METHODS*

Method	Energy (kJ)
Boiled	336
Baked in jacket	357
Mashed (with milk and butter)	504
Roasted	630
Chips	1 050
Crisps	2 226

■ ■ ■

Salads Including a small salad as part of lunch or dinner can help slow down eating and resolve initial hunger. Use a wide selection of vegetables with lower energy values (for examples, see appendix 3) and limit the amount of dressing used. Choose dressings that are low in fat and oil and go a long way. Fresh lemon or orange juice, oil and vinegar dressing, vinegar and tomato juice or red wine dressings. There are several varieties of suitable oil-free dressings available at supermarkets.

Fat and oils Keep these to the barest minimum. No added fat is the best policy. This includes snacks and desserts. Use trim milk, lower fat varieties of foods and minimal fat when required. Butter only one side of the bread, reduce oil added in cooking, keep chocolate, roast meat and roast vegetables for special occasions and limit takeaways. Fat provides the largest number of kilojoules per gram when compared to any other nutrient. A little goes a long way.

Soups Choose light, clear soups without added cereals, cream or butter. If the flavour is strong dilute with trim milk or water. Add vegetables such as celery, cabbage, green beans and tomato rather than legumes and lentils. Rather than eating biscuits and cake, toasted sandwiches or pies, a cup of soup can delay hunger and provide warmth in the winter.

Desserts Choose low fat desserts without added sugar. Fresh fruit makes a suitable alternative. Ice cream is high in fat and sugar so include it only occasionally. Try to increase salad vegetables rather than eating dessert. Use low fat milks and reduce sugar where possible.

Legumes, nuts and seeds These foods are high in carbohydrate and some are very high in fat. Nuts and seeds are often pressed to produce oils. When soya beans or kidney beans are used as the main portion of a meal serve a salad as the accompaniment.

Snacks Eating between meals can provide a significant portion of the daily energy intake. Keep snacks to a minimum. If you miss breakfast, you often feel like a snack around 3-4 p.m., so to avoid this eat regular meals. Choices such as popcorn (without salt and butter), plain wholegrain crackers, fresh fruit or a cup of soup are suitable. Remember, a snack is not a meal. If you are exercising after work or in the middle of the afternoon a light snack may be suitable two hours before activity.

Alcohol The addition of alcohol provides a high intake of energy for very few nutrients. Alcohol also weakens the will-power and more food may be consumed than anticipated. Another concern is the high salt food that is served with alcohol as snacks and nibbles. Increasing salt intake promotes thirst as the body attempts to excrete the added sodium. In social settings this can increase the consumption of alcohol. Water is the preferred fluid. Other suitable alternatives are soda water, diluted fruit juice, soda and lime. Add more ice to alcoholic drinks and drink slowly.

The objective with weight reduction is to choose the most nutrient dense food for the required energy intake — that is, getting more nutrient per slice or serving so performance and training are not compromised.

Menu for weight loss

An intake of 5 MJ (1 200 Cal) for women and 6.3 MJ (1 500 Cal) for men is a guideline for weight reduction programmes, but this depends on individual factors and time frame. Many athletes can lose weight on higher energy intakes. It is necessary to determine the initial total daily intake before any adjustments are made. Then reduce this amount by 2.1 MJ (500 Cal) daily for a total deficit of 14.7 MJ (3 500 Cal) per week. This will promote a loss of 0.5 kg or 1 lb per week.

■ *OUTLINE BREAKFAST*

2 choices bread and cereal group
1 choice fruit and vegetable

1 choice milk and dairy products
1 choice fat

Example: 1 slice thin wholegrain toast (with 1 tsp margarine)
½ cup cereal
1 cup low fat or trim milk
½ cup fresh or stewed fruit (no added sugar)
1 tsp margarine

■ *OUTLINE LUNCH*

2 choices bread and cereal
1 choice meat and alternatives milk
1 choice fruit and vegetable

2 choices low energy vegetables
1 choice fat

Example: 50 g lean meat (no fat or skin)/75 g cottage cheese
2 slices wholegrain bread
1 tsp low-calorie dressing
1 cup salad vegetables
1 orange

■ *OUTLINE DINNER*

2 choices meat and alternatives
3 choices fruit & vegetable or bread & cereal
2 choices low calorie vegetables

Example: 100 g chicken (no skin)
1 baked potato
1 medium carrot
½ cup peas
1 cup cabbage
½ cup popcorn

■ *ANALYSIS*

Energy 6 300 kJ (1 500 Cal)

Carbohydrate	54.5%	202 g
Fat	26.5%	45 g
Protein	19%	76 g

■ ■ ■

For additional options and exchanges, see appendix 3.

16
Health foods and fad diets

No pill, powder, potion or special meal has any magical properties to replace the time and effort put into training and good nutrition.

A great deal of nutrition information is published these days. Some of it is accurate, some not. An American survey in 1982 rated the nutritional information published by several leading women's magazines. Much of the information published in articles in these magazines was evaluated as either inconsistent in terms of accuracy or completely inaccurate.

A fad diet involves a food or drink consumed regularly that is popular or adopted with enthusiasm for a brief period of time, after which it is usually forgotten and replaced by the next phenomenon. This usually produces a cycle of repeated behaviours. There is a regular flow of new fad diets that claim to bring improvements to health, cure illnesses or assist in the slimming process. Pressure to achieve the ideal body weight is felt by many people in today's society. Fad diets promise quick results for minimal effort. These products or diets play upon the hopes, fears and lack of knowledge of individuals.

Exceeding the adequate daily intake is viewed as supernutrition, but supplements can be expensive and are often ineffective. Some are toxic and others can result in nutritional deficiencies. For example, in Zen macrobiotic diets, which are extreme forms of vegetarianism, foods are gradually eliminated until only brown rice is eaten, and fluids are also severely restricted. This type of eating pattern is not suitable for athletes.

Diets such as the Beverly Hills diet, the Mayo Clinic diet, the New York diet and the Chicago diet are based more on geography than balanced eating patterns. Many rely on a common theme, such as raw food, fruit only (the Beverly Hills diet), bread one day and other food the next (the day-on-day-off bread diet), liquid diets, or high protein or high fibre intakes. The Beverly Hills diet and Richard Simmons' 'never-say-diet' diet provide less than 70 percent of the US RDAs (recommended daily allowances) for more than half the vitamins and minerals. The Cambridge diet and other very low energy diets are not suitable for any person actively involved in sports. The carbohydrate content is too low and insufficient energy results in fatigue, which reduces the effectiveness of training and performance.

Promoters claim certain supplements can improve physical performance, reduce weight or treat disease. For athletes seeking drugless ways to obtain a competitive edge, these products may appeal because sometimes the levels are so high in these supplements that they may appear to act like drugs.

Diets based on one food or a limited number of foods lead to nutritional deficiencies and boredom, and do not change eating habits. To achieve a permanent weight loss eating habits must change. Otherwise, like the 'seven day wonder diet', you diet for seven days and then wonder why you gained the weight back!

High protein regimes, such as the 'Scarsdale diet' and 'Dr Atkins' diet revolution', result in bad breath and are inappropriate for people watching dietary intakes of cholesterol. The Atkins diet is also high in fat. As water losses are high these programmes are not recommended for anyone actively involved in sport.

People looking for a competitive edge in sport are often susceptible to advice about various nutritional supplements. This advice may come from a coach or trainer, other athletes or well-meaning onlookers. 'Ergogenic aids' is the term given to substances taken by the athlete or sportsperson in the belief they will improve or enhance strength, performance or endurance. Use of these supplements may be dangerous and rarely improves performance.

The placebo effect

It is relevant to mention the placebo effect when discussing fad diets and supplements. This is defined as any treatment or part of a treatment (such as a diet, food or pill) that does not have a specific action on the consumer's symptoms or disease. The mechanism and

134

effect of a placebo is not well understood. Placebos may work where the illness is emotional; the mind is a powerful tool. If athletes believe taking a particular substance will improve performance, the strength of this belief can be strong enough to result in improved performance. This can occur even if there is no evidence to support a benefit from the product.

Dietary myths

PABA
This substance is called para-amino-benzoic acid and is often listed as a B vitamin. However, it does not meet all the requirements of a vitamin. The body can manufacture PABA as it is needed, so any form of supplementation is unnecessary.

Carnitine
Carnitine has also been called vitamin B$_T$. It is promoted as a new nutrition factor that relieves fatigue and muscle pain in athletes. Under normal conditions there is no requirement for carnitine and for this reason it cannot be considered a vitamin. The role of carnitine in the human body is to enhance the movement of fatty acids into the cells for oxidation. However, supplementing the diet with carnitine has not shown an increase in fatty acid oxidation during exercise. There is no benefit to be gained in taking carnitine to improve sports performance.

Fructose
Fructose is a very simple sugar found mainly in fruits. Forty percent of honey is fructose. Fructose differs slightly from glucose in chemical structure in that it does not require insulin (a hormone which controls blood sugar levels) for absorption into the cells. As a result it does not cause the problems associated with low blood sugars (hypoglycaemia) during exercise. However, if too much fructose is consumed it can cause stomach and intestinal cramps and upsets. Further investigation into the role of fructose in exercise is needed to assess the effects on glycogen sparing and endurance performance.

Wheatgerm and wheatgerm oil
Some coaches and sports participants believe that these substances improve exercise performance, particularly endurance. Thomas Cureton's work in the 1940s and 1950s reported the results of experimental trials and personal observations on the use of

wheatgerm oil. Athletes on wheatgerm oil were said to outperform those on a placebo. Cureton rejected the theory that vitamin E (wheatgerm oil is a very rich source) was responsible. These benefits have never been demonstrated in work by further researchers. The special ingredient found in wheatgerm oil, which is said to benefit sportspeople, has more recently been named octacosanol. This is an alcohol extracted from wheatgerm that, it is alleged, provides energy and enhances performance in endurance events. There is no known ergogenic effect of this substance.

Vitamin E (alpha-tocopherol)

Vitamin E appears important for normal creatine excretion and maintenance of the blood and tissues, but vitamin E deficiencies are extremely rare. It is difficult to eat a diet deficient in this vitamin as it is found in a wide variety of food. In one study on middle distance runners, additional vitamin E failed to show any significant gains in oxygen consumption. It is important to note that no vitamin taken in excess of the ADI has been shown to produce an ergogenic effect.

Carob

This is the fruit of a Mediterranean tree. The powder is obtained by grinding the pods after the seeds are removed. The seed of the carob is the source of a gum used extensively in the food manufacturing industry as a thickener and stabiliser (known as locust bean gum). More recently, carob powder has been promoted as a substitute for cocoa and chocolate products. When comparing cocoa with carob per 100 g, there is little difference in the energy value and mineral content. As carob can be used in some recipes without adding sugar for sweetening the energy value in cooking can be lower. Also, carob does not contain the stimulant theobrimine (similar to caffeine), which is found in cocoa. There is little difference from a nutritional point of view if choosing between carob or chocolate coated sweets and muesli bars.

Bottled water

Bottled water has become very popular in recent years and has followed the increase in diet soda and wine coolers. Initially marketed as a sophisticated drink with high social status, the emphasis has now changed to focus on possible benefits to health. As the population is being encouraged to drink more water the words 'pure', 'natural', 'no calories', 'no added sugar' and 'healthy' readily appear on the labels. There are many varieties of bottled water, including imported and New Zealand-exported lines packaged in plastic, glass bottles or cans. Increase in the use of bottled water might be related to either dissatisfaction with tap water or social affectation rather than any concern for improved health.

However, one cannot argue against the benefits of increasing consumption of water, whatever the form in which it is supplied. Water is essential to life and dehydration rapidly affects sports performance. Also, the health benefits associated with the reduction in the consumption of sugared cordials and soft drinks, beverages and alcohol cannot be ignored. It is important to read the labels, as all bottled water is not created equal. Keep a close eye on the sodium levels particularly with mineral waters.

Brewer's yeast

Many athletes use brewer's yeast in the belief that it is an energy food. Even though it contains a moderate source of B vitamins, there is no evidence that supplementation in this form will benefit sports performance. Brewer's yeast is a by-product of the brewing industry.

Bee pollen

Bee pollen is available in various forms, from pills to powders. Often promoted as nature's miracle food it is believed by coaches and athletes to promote and increase sports performance. Other benefits include correction of digestive problems, resistance to colds and allergies, and improving vitality and energy. Bee pollen is a mixture of bee saliva, plant nectar and pollen. Results of various research studies on runners and swimmers failed to find any benefits. In fact, some sensitive individuals may experience serious allergic reactions.

A similar compound, royal jelly, is produced by worker bees and fed to the queen bee. However, there is no evidence to suggest that either of these substances can enhance performance in humans.

Ginseng

Although claimed at regular intervals to be a sexual enhancer and to act in a similar way to a steroid drug, ginseng and extracts of ginseng have not been shown to have any beneficial effect for sportspeople. There are several side-effects that may arise from excessive intakes of ginseng. These include diarrhoea, nervousness, confusion, depression, and possibly skin eruption and swollen, painful breasts. These effects may impair exercise and performance in some sportspeople.

Amino acid supplements

Amino acids are the building blocks of protein and keen interest is developing in using large doses of individual amino acids as a supplement. It has been suggested that specific amino acids taken in this way may stimulate growth hormone production and thereby promote muscle growth. Two proteins that have been promoted as enhancing strength or endurance are glycine and gelatin. Neither provide any improvement to performance. Bodybuilders are common users of these supplements, believing they aid the recovery of muscle after weightlifting. However, scientific evidence to support these claims is in short supply.

Protein supplements

When muscle is viewed as the key to performance, the concept of the more muscle the better prevails, and any method claiming to promote a rapid increase in this tissue may be welcomed. A popular belief held by coaches and athletes is that amino acids and protein supplements stimulate growth. However, it is important to remember that muscle growth is stimulated by exercise. The type of exercise required is highly intensive, using 70 percent of maximum output, which increases the tension on the muscle (for example, weightlifting exercises). The resulting muscle growth is due to increased protein synthesis (buildup) or decreased protein breakdown.

Supplements vary greatly in the amount of protein they provide. One protein tablet may contain up to 1-2 g of protein, and two tablespoons of a protein powder varies in protein content from 5 g to 10 g, depending on whether the drink is made with water or milk. It is difficult to imagine a New Zealand diet that is deficient in protein, so it should not be necessary to supplement. Eating a balanced diet can provide sufficient and in most cases additional protein.

There are some problems associated with consuming excessive protein; these include dehydration, gout and urinary losses of calcium. Remember that if the additional protein is not required for muscle synthesis it is converted to fat and stored by the body.

Choline

Choline is more commonly recognised as lecithin (its main dietary source) and it is present in the brain and other nerve tissues. Promoters claim choline can improve or cure mental disorders, improve memory, and mobilise fat and cholesterol from the liver. The human requirement for choline has not been identified. It does not meet the definition of a vitamin, although some attempts have been made to give it B vitamin status. Lecithin is promoted as a cure for high cholesterol levels. However, there is no good evidence to suggest this is a benefit to humans. Lecithin does not promote weight loss when consumed on its own or mixed with cider vinegar, kelp or vitamin supplements. It is widely spread amongst foods and a balanced, varied diet appears to provide sufficient intake. Food sources include egg yolk, organ meats, whole grains, cereals and legumes. It is used heavily in the manufacturing industry as an emulsifier. At 20 times normal intakes such side-effects as nausea, dizziness, diarrhoea, heart disturbances and a fish-like odour have been reported. As no benefits have been reported, sports participants can gain no advantage from increased intakes of lecithin.

Pangamic acid

Pangamic acid, or vitamin B_{15}, is often advertised as a vitamin that increases the delivery of oxygen to cells and tissues. This substance, obtained from apricot kernels, bitter almonds, and peach and apple seeds, has never been shown to have any recognised vitamin function; therefore, it cannot be classified as a vitamin. Sportspeople have claimed the use of pangamic acid has improved physical performance. However, this may have been due to the placebo effect, as studies have shown no change in oxygen consumption during controlled tests.

The composition of these tablets varies widely. The analysis of one variety was found to contain pure lactose (milk sugar). Another substance, often called B_{15}, is laetril, which was once promoted as a cancer remedy. It contains 6 percent cyanide by weight and releases the cyanide when broken down within the digestive system. There is no evidence to suggest that this is effective against cancer.

Spirulina

A newer product being promoted through so-called health food stores is a microscopic blue-green alga called spirulina. Potentially toxic, this has limited benefit nutritionally and is contaminated with bacteria and insect debris. This product does not provide any benefit to sports performance.

Health foods

The term 'health food' is used to describe 'natural' or 'organic' foods. Generally these are foods that have received less processing or refining compared with other foods. Examples are wholegrain cereals, wholemeal flour and whole foods such as seeds and nuts.

Many everyday foods have taken on 'health food' status. These include honey, some varieties of oils, raw sugar, many vegetarian foods (soya bean-based products), rock salt, sea salt and some beverages (herbal teas). Certain foods, marketed as healthy snacks, such as some fruit bars and muesli bars, can only be called candy, because of the amount of sugar added in the form of honey, malt and glucose. A healthy diet should contain a wide variety of foods. There is no one perfect food, neither does any one food hold special properties.

Organic foods are generally plant foods grown without the use of chemical fertilisers or pesticides. Animals that have been fed un-processed foods are also included. Organic foods are also processed without any 'artificial' ingredients. However, because of the risk of food poisoning from bacteria, which are present in animal-based composts used for fertiliser, it is very important than any uncooked food is washed throughly. There is no evidence to suggest that organic foods are nutritionally superior.

The Pritikin diet

This diet is high in complex carbohydrates (whole grains, fruits, vegetables and legumes), low in cholesterol, contains less than 10 percent fat and is low in protein. The original purpose of this diet was to aid those with heart disease and individuals with elevated fat and cholesterol levels in the blood. Pritikin believed that his diet could reverse hardening of the arteries (atherosclerosis). Caffeine-containing beverages such as tea and coffee are excluded from the diet, as is alcohol.

Though high in carbohydrate and fibre, the diet is extreme for athletes. There is no evidence that food such as eggs, nuts, cheese or low fat dairy products should be excluded and this would place calcium intake at risk. Fat and sodium deficiencies have been reported on this diet. In addition, the diet is low in iron and zinc.

Concern has been expressed about the energy content in the bulky food in the Pritikin diet. Some athletes who follow this diet to the extreme may compromise their energy levels. Some may also experience discomfort from bulky bowels during intense endurance activity. Excessive fibre interferes with calcium and the absorption of other minerals. Bloating, flatulence, abdominal pain and diarrhoea can result if the amount of recommended fibre is not added to the eating pattern gradually. A modified, more flexible version that in-cludes more protein, iron and zinc while maintaining lower fat, sugar, salt and alcohol levels is more appropriate for athletes.

Fad diets

Sportspeople are under a lot of pressure to reduce weight so as to have a leaner, stronger or lighter body, or to be able to move faster.

Dieting has a negative image and many people, including athletes, see it as a hassle. Many look for quick, magic, no hassle, dramatic programmes.

The following table rates some of the more popular diets on the basis of whether they contain the necessary criteria for success. These criteria are:

Safety Is the diet nutritionally safe, without harmful side-effects to health or nutritional status?

Ease Is the diet easy to use, convenient and requiring minimal skill? Are dishes simple to prepare and are ingredients familiar and readily accessible?

Family application Can the whole family enjoy the meals? If so, there will be no need for separate cooking and purchasing patterns.

Cost Is the diet expensive or does it involve minimal or no additional cost?

Variety Does the diet contain a wide selection of foods? Eating the same food in a repetitive pattern induces boredom and limits compliance and flexibility.

Suitability Is this eating pattern suitable for people actively engaged in sports activity? Is there a possibility of a detrimental effect on performance?

■ DIET RATINGS

CODE Y/N=depends on circumstances, E=expensive, R=reasonable cost, M=minimal or no additional cost.

Diet	Safe	Ease	Family	Cost	Variety	Suitable
Beverly Hills	No	No	No	E	No	No

Comments Involves fruit only. Some foods are difficult to obtain. Unsuitable for children and athletes.

Diet	Safety	Ease	Family	Cost	Variety	Suitable
Cambridge	No	No	No	R	Yes	No

Comments Very low calorie diet. Unsuitable for the active or children.

Diet	Safe	Ease	Family	Cost	Variety	Suitable
Very Low Energy	No	Yes	No	R	No	No

Comments Should only be used for a short time. Low in carbohydrate. Can be expensive.

Diet	Safe	Ease	Family	Cost	Variety	Suitable
Atkins	No	No	No	R	Yes	No

Comments High fat/low carbohydrate intakes induce ketosis. Excessive fat intake contradicts New Zealand nutritional recommendations. Can be expensive with high meat consumption. Causes significant loss of lean muscle tissue.

Diet	Safe	Ease	Family	Cost	Variety	Suitable
Scarsdale	Yes	Y/N	Y/N	R	No	No

Comments For two weeks separate meals are prepared, which are low in carbohydrate and high in protein. Iron and calcium intakes are limited. Not recommended.

Diet	Safe	Ease	Family	Cost	Variety	Suitable
Grapefruit	No	Yes	No	M	No	No

Comments Eating grapefruit before each meal can be monotonous. Meals are low carbohydrate, high protein, high fat. Grapefruits have no special powers to break down or burn fat.

Diet	Safe	Ease	Family	Cost	Variety	Suitable
Never-say-diet	Yes	Yes	Y/N	R	Yes	Y/N

Comments Involves reduced calories. Generally not suitable for children and active adults.

Diet	Safe	Ease	Family	Cost	Variety	Suitable
Hip and Thigh	Yes	Yes	No	R	Yes	Y/N

Comments Basically a low fat diet. It is not possible to reduce weight from specific parts of the body. Weight loss will occur from all over the body and exercise will change the shape of certain areas. Not recommended for children or active athletes.

Diet	Safe	Ease	Family	Cost	Variety	Suitable
Liquid	No	Yes	No	E	No	No

Comments Usually high in protein and low in carbohydrate content. Insufficient energy for active individuals. Rapid weight loss can be hazardous (some deaths have occurred as a result of low potassium levels). Refrigeration is necessary if liquid food mixed in bulk. Unpalatable for some.

Diet	Safe	Ease	Family	Cost	Variety	Suitable
Fasting	No	No	No	M	No	No

Comments With only water or diluted fruit juice, fasting is totally inappropriate for athletes. This regime has been used for short periods of time when individuals are under strict medical supervision. Though effective, there are numerous side-effects. The brain uses large amounts of glucose. When glucose is in short supply an alternative fuel, ketone bodies, supplies the brain with energy. This is called ketosis. Some form of carbohydrate is necessary to prevent this from occurring.

■ ■ ■

17
Vegetarian eating patterns

Vegetarian eating patterns are more popular now than they were in the past. Among the reasons for this change in eating patterns are a concern for animals, a dislike of red meat and a desire for improved health and nutritional status. In *Nutritional Guidelines for New Zealanders* (see Bibliography), one of the recommendations is that more vegetarian meals be included in the general eating pattern.

A sportsperson can perform well on a vegetarian or meatless food pattern. However, becoming a vegetarian involves more than simply cutting out all forms of red meat; there are several different levels of vegetarianism.

A number of health benefits can be gained from switching to this type of eating pattern. Research has shown that vegetarians, as a group, have lower blood fat levels, less heart disease and are less prone to certain types of cancer than the general population. A vegetarian diet can also relieve problems of constipation and excess weight because of its high fibre content.

A vegetarian eating pattern lowers fat intake because of the reduction in consumption of red meat and full cream dairy products. The higher intake of cereals, fruit and vegetables provides considerably more fibre. However, a vegetarian food plan for sports performance must include adequate quantities of all the essential nutrients. Of particular importance are the essential amino acids, folate, vitamin B_{12}, iron, calcium and zinc. Legumes are a good source of all B vitamins except riboflavin and vitamin B_{12}. They also provide fibre and some minerals. But, compared to meat, legumes are not a good source of the minerals iron, copper and zinc. Sprouted beans are an excellent source of vitamin C.

Obtaining sufficient energy may sometimes be difficult with this diet. Athletes may have to struggle to get enough food of a bulky nature. Fructarian (only fruit), grainarian (only grains) or macrobiotic diets are examples of extreme vegetarian diets that do not provide a balanced intake of nutrients, particularly energy, for an individual involved in sport.

Types of vegetarianism

Vegetarians follow eating patterns in which animal products, such as meat, fish and chicken, are replaced with plant foods, such as fruit, nuts, cereals and vegetables. There are three main categories of vegetarians and each is based on a different variation of this main theme.

Lacto ovo vegetarian   Lacto refers to milk and ovo to eggs. Hence, a lacto ovo vegetarian (or ovo lactarian) is a person who will consume milk, milk products and eggs but no other animal products in addition to plant foods.

Lacto vegetarian   These vegetarians do not eat eggs or meat. However, milk products are eaten in addition to plant foods.

Vegan   A vegan is a stricter form of vegetarian. No animal products are eaten. Much reliance is placed on obtaining a balanced diet from combining various cereal and plant foods. A strict vegan diet must be carefully planned to avoid deficiencies in protein, vitamin and minerals in the long term.

Semi-vegetarian   This is a possible fourth classification, which identifies people who consume some animal foods but, generally, exclude red meat. For example, fish and chicken may be eaten, in addition to dairy products, cereals and plant foods.

Achieving a balanced diet

Two important factors to consider in a vegetarian eating pattern are *quality* and *quantity*. To obtain a balance of proteins, it is important for vegetarians to eat a wide variety of food. Proteins are made up of smaller units called amino acids, which build and maintain the muscle, tissues, enzymes and many other substances in the body.

145

There are eight essential amino acids for adults and 10 for children. Dietary protein must supply all the essential amino acids as the body is unable to produce these. Animal and vegetable protein differ in the quality and quantity of the essential amino acids.

The inclusion of dairy products and eggs assists sports participants to achieve a balanced vegetarian diet, as both milk and eggs contain all the essential amino acids required for health. These foods are also good sources of calcium, riboflavin, and vitamins A, D and B_{12}. Care must be taken with vegetarian diets because, unlike animal foods, plant foods generally do not contain all the essential amino acids in one food. Cereals are low in the amino acid lysine; and beans are low in the amino acid methionine, though rich in lysine.

■ QUALITY OF DIFFERENT PROTEIN FOODS

Food	Protein quality — limiting amino acid
Milk	complete
Cheese (cottage, cheddar)	complete
Yoghurt	complete
Meat, fish, poultry	complete
Eggs	complete
Dried beans, peas	incomplete — methionine
Lentils	incomplete — methionine
Peanut butter	incomplete — several borderline
Breakfast cereals (wheat)	incomplete — lysine
Breakfast cereals (corn)	incomplete — lysine, tryptophan
Spaghetti, macaroni	incomplete — lysine
Rice	incomplete — lysine, threonine
Bread	incomplete — lysine
Brewer's yeast	borderline — methionine

■ ■ ■

The term 'limiting amino acid' is given to the amino acid that is found to be low or absent in a food. Vegetables alone do not provide a balanced meal. Plant foods must be combined to provide these essential amino acids and ensure a sufficient supply of high quality protein. This can sometimes be done in a single dish; for example, combine cereals and vegetables with milk (macaroni cheese) or legumes (dried beans, peas, soya beans) with cereals (rice). Increase the frequency of soya beans and chick peas, or other vegetables that are high in protein. Compared to other beans, soya beans contain twice the protein, four times the fat and one-third the carbohydrate.

146

Vegetarian food groups

Foods from each of the following groups should be combined to provide a balance of amino acids.

Grains Rice (raw, white or brown), tortillas, corn, oatmeal bread, pasta, breakfast cereals.

Seeds and nuts Pumpkin, sesame and sunflower seeds, walnuts, almonds, brazil nuts, cashews, hazelnuts, pine nuts, peanuts and peanut butter, pistachios.

Milk products and eggs Milk, cheese, yoghurt.

Legumes Split peas, chickpeas, dried beans, kidney beans, baked beans, lima beans, haricot beans, mung beans, soya beans, broad beans, pinto beans, lentils.

Examples of dishes that combine complementary protein groups, which will provide all the essential amino acids, are stuffed vegetables, spinach soufflé, vegetables with cheese sauces, savoury omelettes, pasta with toppings, and mixed grains. The following list provide ideas for dishes that combine two food groups.

Grain plus milk products Rice and milk (rice pudding or baked savoury), bread with cheese and milk, macaroni cheese, cheese or egg sandwiches, pasta and egg salad, eggs on toast, spaghetti with grated cheese, porridge and milk.

Grain plus seeds and nuts Rice and nut casserole, peanut butter sandwich, rice and walnut salad, corn and peanuts, pasta and seeds, spaghetti and nut sauce, muesli, seeds and nuts sprinkled over rice salad or rice pudding.

Grain plus legumes Rice and bean casserole, risotto with beans and vegetables, lentil curry and rice, wheat bread and baked beans, pea soup and toast, pasta with bean and vegetable sauce, chickpea dip and unleavened bread (Lebanese), lentil purée and rice (Indian), corn tortilla and chilli beans (Mexican), soya beans and rice, pea soup and cornbread.

Legumes plus seeds and nuts Sesame seeds in bean casserole, sunflower seeds and peanuts, legume soup and bread, sesame seeds and chick peas.

147

Legumes plus milk products Milk with bean soup, cheese sauce on beans, beans and eggs.

Milk products plus seeds and nuts Sesame seeds and cheese sauce, peanuts and eggs.

Baseline vegetarian food plan

Selecting any three servings of the following foods each day will assist in providing an adequate intake of protein.

Food	Serving	Protein g
Milk	300 ml	10
Milk (children)	600 ml	20
Cheese	50 g	12
Cottage cheese	½ cup	12
Yoghurt	1 cup	12
Eggs	2	12
Bread (wholegrain)	4 slices	12
Breakfast cereals	60 g	7
Pasta uncooked	55 g	7
Oatmeal uncooked	60 g	8
Corn tortillas	3	7
Rice	60 g	4
Beans dried	75 g	5
Beans cooked/canned	175 g	10
Baked beans	175–200 g	10
Lentils/split peas	65 g	5
Nuts/seeds	40–50 g	11
Peanut butter	35 g	10

■ ■ ■

At least four servings of fruit, vegetables, sprouts and juices should be eaten daily. This is not usually difficult for vegetarians.

The nutritional guidelines for sportspeople also apply to the vegetarian and there are several areas that require particular attention by the vegetarian involved in sport. Vegetarians must take particular care to obtain adequate vitamin B_2 (riboflavin), vitamin B_{12}, vitamin D, iron, calcium and zinc. Vitamin B_2, vitamin D and calcium are especially important considerations for vegans because no dairy products are consumed. However, margarine contains added vitamin D and, with exposure to sunlight, it is unlikely that the vegan's diet will be deficient in this vitamin. To obtain adequate B_2, increase the regular intake of green vegetables, yeast extracts, cereals and nuts.

Pregnancy and breastfeeding also place extra demands for B_{12} and a vitamin B_{12} supplement may be recommended under these conditions. Vitamin B_{12} is not found in plant foods unless the food has been fermented or contains bacteria. The soya bean product tempeh and mushrooms both contain vitamin B_{12}. Vitamin B_{12} is stored in the liver for 3–5 years so deficiencies take a considerable time to develop.

Including soya milk will provide extra calcium, as will nuts (cashew), sesame seeds, legumes (soya bean) and green-leaf vegetables. Green-leaf vegetables are also good sources of iron, which is generally poorly absorbed. Although around 10 percent of iron found in meat is absorbed, less than 5 percent is available from non-meat sources. Anaemia from iron deficiency is a common problem for vegetarians, particularly for women. A vegetarian can obtain zinc from wholegrain cereals.

Young adults and children

Strict vegetarian diets may place the health of young children at risk for several reasons. A vegetarian diet is high in fibre and children may find it difficult to consume enough food to provide sufficient energy for growth. The inclusion of milk will relieve this problem. Foods can be chopped to facilitate digestion and a few higher energy snacks can be added (such as cheese, honey, eggs and oils). A vegetarian diet introduced too soon into an infant food plan may cause problems with digestion as the gastrointestinal tract is too immature to handle the bulky nature of the food. Introduce weaning foods gradually. For the young sportsperson, ensure that adequate energy, iron, calcium and vitamin B_{12} are consumed to cater for growth and the additional demands of exercise.

■ EXAMPLE OF A BALANCED VEGETARIAN MENU

Breakfast
Fruit x 2	1 glass orange juice
Bread x 4	2 Weetbix + 2 wholegrain toast
Milk x 1	1 glass trim milk
Fat x 2	2 tbsp peanut butter

Lunch
Bread x 2	2 slices wholegrain bread or 1 large pita bread
Vegetables x 3	1 large cup vegetable salad
Milk x 1	½ cup cottage cheese or 50 g cheddar cheese
Fat x 2	2 tsp margarine
Fruit x 3	apple, large banana and ½ cup pineapple juice

Dinner

Bread x 4	½ small low fat pizza and 1 baked potato with cheese
Vegetables x 2	1 large cup salad
Fat x 2	2 tbsp oil and vinegar dressing
Fruit x 1	1 nectarine
Milk x 1	1 cup natural low fat yoghurt
Fruit x 1	½ cup strawberries
Bread x 1	¼ cup muesli (low fat)

Snacks

Fruit x 3	1 orange, 3 dates, 7–8 dried apricots
Bread x 1	3 crackers
Fat x 1	1 tbsp unsalted peanuts (20)

Analysis

Energy 12.6 MJ	3 000 Cal
CHO 65%	481 g
Fat 24%	81 g
Protein 11%	90 g
Iron	19 mg

See appendix 3 for a range of alternatives.

■ ■ ■

18
Pre-competition food

Once the baseline eating patterns are firmly established and the training meals are well refined, the third phase, examining the pre-event meals, becomes possible.

When to eat

The pre-event meal provides the athlete with sufficient food energy and optimum hydration for the event or game. It is important to allow sufficient time for this food to be digested. High fat foods should be eliminated because they are slow to be digested. These should be replaced with carbohydrate foods. It is preferable to eat 2–3 hours before an event, but this time frame varies according to each individual. The increased tension generally associated with competitive events or games reduces the blood flow to the digestive system, decreasing the rate of digestion.

There are several reasons why food should not be eaten immediately before exercise. During exercise, the body uses the stores of muscle glycogen and body fat. Any food consumed immediately before activity will not increase these stores. When exercising, blood that has been directed to the digestive system is redirected to the exercising muscle. This slows down digestion and the food remains in the stomach. As a result, some people who exercise after eating feel nauseated, distended in the stomach and uncomfortable. This may also restrict breathing.

151

If food is to be eaten it should be low fat, low protein and high in carbohydrates. A light snack a few hours beforehand will ward off feelings of hunger.

What to eat

Foods included in pre-event meals should be easily digested, provide energy and fluid, and be familiar and enjoyable. The size of meals may vary according to appetite. Commercially prepared liquid meals are suitable because they are high in carbohydrate and contain adequate amounts of fat and protein to promote feelings of fullness and delay the onset of hunger. In addition, they are easily digested and leave minimal residue in the digestive tract. Ensure or Sustagen are two possibilities for the athlete who, through nervousness, finds it difficult to eat solid food. Made with water or trim milk they provide a low fat alternative. Care must be taken to follow instructions on rehydrating the formula, so as to avoid excesses that may interfere with performance.

Nothing new should be tried on the day of the event. Test all meals and procedures beforehand during training. There is no room for the unexpected on the day of the event.

Many sportspeople believe a high sugar snack or glucose supplement just before competition will help their performance. But a pre-event snack that is high in sugar increases the rate of glycogen use by the muscle. As sugar enters the blood, the rapidly rising blood glucose levels cause an increase in insulin. This insulin inhibits the use of fatty acids for fuel, and the body must then rely on muscle glycogen and the blood glucose for energy. (For a detailed account of the effect of sugar and glucose on sports performance, see chapter 4.)

Reports on the ingestion of sucrose, glucose or glucose polymer solution during events indicate these may have a glycogen sparing effect and improve endurance in events of two hours or more. However, the initial muscle glycogen stores built up before exercise are important to endurance; consuming carbohydrate drinks may not have a significant advantage if these stores are already loaded at the onset of exercise.

For any activity lasting under 2 hours water is the preferred liquid. Any liquid containing sugar or glucose must be diluted to 2.5 g per 100 ml and consumed up to 1 hour before performance. Some diluted vegetable juices may be a suitable alternative, but care must be taken with the sodium content. Fruit juices should also be diluted. For events lasting longer than 2 hours, such as the Ironman or Coast-to-coast, special considerations apply. (See chapter 19.) The competitor must consume adequate fluid to ensure that he or she is fully hydrated before commencing any sports event.

As well as fluids, the pre-event meal may include carbohydrate loading, especially for ultra endurance events. Performance can be significantly impaired with poor eating practices. Take care with foods that are high in fibre content, as these can cause flatulence (wind) and can result in discomfort during exercise if eaten in excessive amounts.

Eat at least 2–3 hours before the event. The pre-event meal should be light and easily digested, low in fat, composed mainly of complex carbohydrates, and include adequate fluids. Food eaten at this time will contribute only a small amount to the demands of the activity, but it will promote hydration.

■ EXAMPLES OF PRE-COMPETITION MEALS

Breakfast
Rice bubbles or cornflakes
Trim or low fat milk
Fruit, fresh or stewed
Toast, light grain or white, with very light
    butter and honey or jam
Fruit juice (diluted)

Lunch

Menu 1
Grilled chicken
Baked potato, rice or pasta
    (hot or as a salad)
Green vegetables or salad
Vegetable soup
Fresh fruit

Menu 2
Low fat pizza
Salad
Fresh fruit
Fruit juice

Menu 3
Filled rolls
Crackers or biscuits
Fresh fruit
Fruit juice

Menu 4
Fresh fruit salad
Soup
Low fat yoghurt
Fruit juice

■ ■ ■

Carbohydrate loading

Sporting activities place heavy demands on muscles and muscle glycogen. Low levels of glycogen in muscle can significantly impair performance.

Early evidence demonstrating an effect of muscle glycogen on sports performance came from studies showing a relationship between the time taken to run 30 km and the level of muscle glycogen at the onset of the activity. The running time was reduced on a high carbohydrate diet as throughout the run optimal speed could be maintained.

Studies on team sports, such as soccer, showed that by half time players who had had a low glycogen level at the start of a match had almost no glycogen remaining in the muscle used, and had covered 25 percent less distance, sprinted less and walked more. All players had very low glycogen levels at the end of the match.

Fatigued sports participants are more likely to make mistakes, lose concentration and receive injuries. It has been suggested that low or depleted glycogen levels may explain accidents, fatigue and unexpected poor sports performance. Many athletes continue to train hard right up until the last minute, utilising glycogen and reducing glycogen stores. Some sportspeople (weightlifters, bodybuilders, wrestlers and jockeys) even limit their intake of carbohydrates and continue intense training to reduce body weight before competition. This behaviour has a negative effect on performance.

Muscle glycogen depletion during exercise depends on the intensity and duration of activity, the diet, the muscle used, and the aerobic capacity of the sports participant. More protein is metabolised for energy in athletes who are glycogen depleted, compared to those with adequate reserves of glycogen. Fatigue occurs when the muscle glycogen falls to a level where the exercise rate can no longer be maintained. In low intensity exercise (walking) the glycogen stores are depleted less quickly.

Glycogen is the major fuel burned at the onset of exercise (during a 1-hour run), once the initial stores of ATP are used up. The liver is the major site of glucose production. For long-term activity, muscle glycogen stores and fat are necessary. Fat assumes a more important role when the carbohydrate reserves are lowered, at the end of activity. The use of fat reduces the use of glycogen and delays exhaustion. In prolonged exercise, when muscle glycogen stores have been used up, the sports participant must reduce the intensity of the exercise because fat oxidation (burning fat for fuel and energy) cannot meet the energy requirements of high intensity exercise. Nevertheless, the body does have the ability to burn fat and protein (as fatty acids and amino acids) to produce fuel for exercise.

To optimise sports performance, both training and correct eating patterns are important factors. Training improves the body's ability to burn fat for fuel, hence sparing carbohydrate reserves in the muscle, and eating the correct food provides the body with the necessary

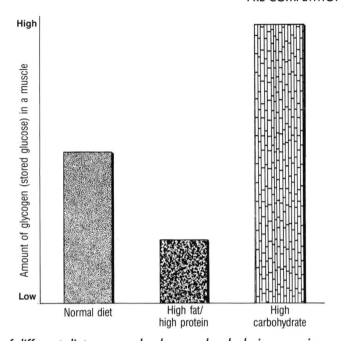

Effects of different diets on muscle glycogen levels during exercise.

(Adapted from Bergstrom et al. Diet, Muscle Glycogen and Physical Performance. *Acta Physiol. Scand.*, 71: 140–150, 1967.)

fuel source. Carbohydrates are the primary fuel source for exercise.

Glycogen, which is in limited supply, is conserved by the body and more fat is used as fuel in endurance events. Carbohydrate loading will not assist an athlete to run faster, only to run for longer before tiring. Even with increased glycogen stores the extra energy will only last for 2-3 hours of intense exercise and it can take several days to restore the depleted muscle glycogen levels.

The glucose and glycogen stored in the blood and tissues supplies sufficient fuel for a healthy individual to perform light activities for about half a day. Hence, more active individuals or trained sports participants need to take some form of carbohydrate at regular intervals throughout a day's training or event. Active, trained athletes also have the ability to store more glycogen than non-active people. Adequate carbohydrate intakes are important to maintain liver glycogen.

Glycogen supercompensation

By making some changes to the basic diet the normal levels of glycogen stored in the muscle and liver can be increased by two to three times the normal amount. High intensity exercise can be

155

maintained for a longer period of time on a high carbohydrate diet of 660 g per day. (Normal levels are approximately 350 g per day.) Complex carbohydrates provide greater glycogen storage than simple sugars. The depletion of glycogen occurs specifically in the muscles used for exercise. For example, cyclists deplete glycogen stores in the quadriceps first.

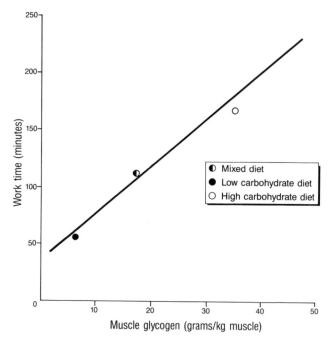

Muscle glycogen loading procedures.

(Adapted from Saltin, B., and Hermansen, L. Glycogen stores and prolonged severe exercise. In Blix, G. (ed). *Nutrition and Physical Activity.* Uppsala, Sweden, 1967.)

The elevation of muscle glycogen stores beyond normal levels is termed **supercompensation**. There are two methods of dietary manipulation used to boost glycogen stores. To be effective, it must be remembered that supercompensation is used only in endurance events, where continuous activity lasts more than 2 hours. It is not suitable for periods of short activity or exercise lasting less than 1 hour.

The classical method requires the glycogen stores to be depleted or emptied by exercise plus a very low carbohydrate diet for three days. Three days before competition a high intake of over 600 g of carbohydrates (60–70 percent) is cosnsumed while the athlete rests. This elevates muscle glycogen levels to almost twice normal levels.

There are some disadvantages to this method. While muscle glycogen is being depleted in the early phase, maintaining adequate intakes of energy is extremely difficult. Weight loss (largely as a result of water and salt excretion), ketosis (a response to mild starvation) and mental and physical fatigue occur. Athletes become irritable and their confidence in their ability is often reduced because of impaired sports performance during training. With the repletion phase of high carbohydrate intake, weight rapidly rises as the water and glycogen are replaced. (3 g of water is stored for every gram of glycogen.) Feelings of stiffness and heaviness are common complaints. Discomforts can be severe enough to cause withdrawal from competition. This method is not recommended for diabetics, young athletes or those at risk of cardiovascular disease. As a result of these difficulties a modified method was devised.

This second method, known as the modern method, maintains the loader on a normal diet (50 percent carbohydrate) for up to 3 days before competition. The diet is then changed to a high carbohydrate intake (60–70 percent), and training is reduced. The method produces similar levels of glycogen storage without the severe dieting and side-effects.

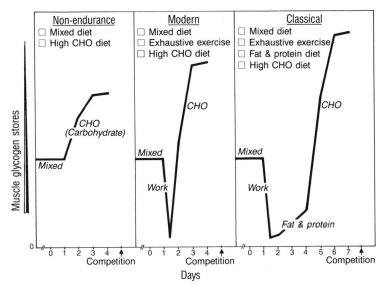

Changes in muscle glycogen levels with exercise.

(Adapted from Costill, D. L., et al. Muscle Glycogen Utilization during Prolonged Exercise on Successive Days. *J. Appl. Physiol.*, 31: 835, 1971.)

Regular training causes some depletion of muscle glycogen stores. With repeated days of heavy training glycogen used can temporarily exceed replacement. This can be easily overcome by eating high carbohydrate meals (65–70 percent) and performing short intense workouts or long easy exercise sessions. This procedure will optimise glycogen replacement, storage and use. Carbohydrate loading is only effective if used two to three times a year.

Foods for carbohydrate loading

The objective of carbohydrate loading is to increase the storage of glycogen in the muscle. Glycogen is the primary source of fuel in endurance events such as marathons, cross-country skiing, distance cycling and swimming. It is not suitable for short events or where flexibility is important, as water stored with the glycogen can make the muscle feel tight and uncomfortable.

Carbohydrate loading is not overeating. Overall food intake does not increase, only the proportion of carbohydrate in the daily intake changes. This means that the loader must reduce the fat and protein content. Include more foods from the bread and cereal food group and the fruit and vegetable food groups. It may be necessary to increase the amount of sugar, honey or foods containing sugar to elevate the carbohydrate content so as to avoid an excessive increase in the bulk of food eaten. The meals should consist of a variety of foods that are pleasant to eat.

■ EXAMPLE OF A MENU FOR CARBOHYDRATE LOADING

Breakfast
1 glass fruit juice (not tomato)
1 cup cereal
1 large banana
½ cup low fat milk
2 toast or an English muffin
2 tsp jam or honey

Lunch
2 chicken Vogels sandwiches (4 bread and two slices chicken)
1 glass fruit juice
2 pieces fruit
1 fruit muffin
2 tsp jam or honey

Dinner
1 cup spaghetti or rice
1 cup savoury tomato topping
grated cheese (1 tbsp parmesan or 2 tbsp grated low fat cheese)
2 slices bread or 1 bread roll
1–2 cups fresh fruit salad or rice pudding

Snacks
1 fruit
½ cup raisins
1 glass fruit juice

Additional snacks according to appetite.
Nutritional analysis

Energy:	12.3 MJ	3 000 Cal
CHO	80%	581 g
Fat	10%	32 g
Protein	10%	81 g

■ ■ ■

The night before an event, be very careful when you choose pasta. This food is often served with rich creamy cheese sauces or swimming in oil. Choose baked potatoes instead of roast potatoes or fried chips, and light spaghetti sauces. Take care with macaroni cheese and pizza which are often covered with cheese. Choose lean meats, such as chicken (no skin), or fish (no batter) and vegetables. Potatoes, pumpkin, kumara, peas, broad beans and parsnips are fine. Drink plenty of fluids.

■ MEALS FOR THE NIGHT BEFORE AN EVENT

2-3 slices low fat pizza with salad (oil and vinegar dressing), or
2 cups spaghetti with tomato topping and 3 slices bread, or
1 cup chicken with 3 baked potatoes, peas and kumara, or
2 cups rice with ½ cup grilled diced meat or lean mince.
Add Salad and other vegetables (especially green leaf vegetables) and fruit, fruit salad, biscuit, yoghurt as required, and drink sufficient fluids.

■ ■ ■

19
Food during events

On the day of the game, event or race, follow the usual eating patterns and do not attempt to try anything new. Don't fall into the trap of thinking that what someone else is eating may be better. You know what works for you, and you have spent weeks or months preparing to compete at peak performance.

Only familiar foods should be eaten. Do not attempt any new, unusual or different foods as this could end in poor performance. Avoid fatty foods, foods with high sugar contents, large amounts of salt, and large volumes of food. Eat a light meal 2–3 hours before the event (see chapter 18) and drink plenty of fluids.

Fluids

Some events, such as the Ironman, Coast-to-coast and other ultra-endurance events, require special attention. Fluids and some form of carbohydrate are important elements in the race plan. Providing the body with an adequate intake of fluid is absolutely essential for any athlete competing in these types of events.

To avoid fatigue and the effects of dehydration, and to enable the athlete to continue, fluid lost during exercise must be replaced. For events under 1–2 hours, water is fine. Events lasting longer will require some carbohydrate replacement. For triathletes, eating on the bike leg is the best solution. Some marathon runners are able to eat sandwiches and continue running.

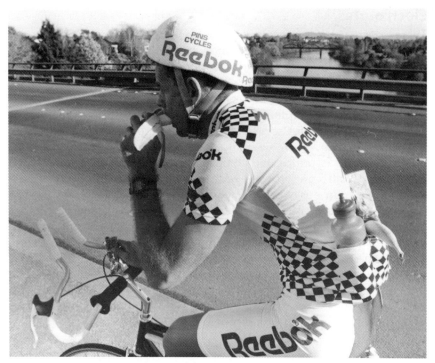

Eating and drinking during events requires practice.

Glycogen replacement

During a long endurance event involving more than 2 hours of continuous activity there is a possibility of glycogen depletion. To delay this, add energy in the form of glucose or glucose polymers (polycose). Glucose polymers contain more energy per gram than glucose without raising the osmotic concentration. Therefore, a higher energy content can be obtained without the adverse effects experienced with a similar concentration of sugar. Diluting fruit juice is another suitable alternative.

There are several sports drinks being marketed in New Zealand as suitable for long events. Many, however, contain excessive quantities of glucose or concentrations of electrolytes that are too high. Solutions high in sugar are slow to leave the stomach and therefore do not provide protection against dehydration. Before using any type of energy replacement fluids check with a sports-medicine doctor or sports nutritionist. Experiment with the solution during training. Stomach cramps and nausea are common side-effects. Diarrhoea may result if the sugar concentration is too high.

Electrolytes

There is no need for electrolyte replacement during most events, despite losses of sodium and chloride caused by sweating. Electrolyte replacement solutions also contain potassium and magnesium and they are more suitable for the recovery phase.

During exercise the kidney retains more of these substances and less is excreted in the urine. Generally, the purpose of the electrolytes present in commercial sports drinks is to increase fluid absorption, not to replace losses in sweating. These solutions are not required unless exercise is performed for prolonged periods in hot climates; for example, ultra-endurance events and ultra-marathons.

Salt losses can easily be replaced by the post-exercise meal, when you can use more salt in or on food, or eat foods containing more salt. Electrolyte supplements during an event can result in fluid retention in the stomach and intestines. Salt tablets must not be taken. These tablets increase the work of the kidneys, can cause nausea and vomiting and, if water intake is limited or reduced, result in dehydration. A varied intake of a wide range of foods supplies the body with more than sufficient salt and electrolytes. Any losses can be easily replaced through normal intakes of food.

Commercial liquid foods

There are several products available at gyms, sports clubs and chemists which provide a range of nutrients and simply require the addition of water or milk, according to the manufacturer's instructions. Let's examine a few of these in closer detail.

Electrolyte replacement drinks

When commercial sports drinks and water are compared, both appear equally effective in maintaining the water and mineral balance. In other words, these replacement solutions provide no advantage over water, and any extra minerals are generally excreted.

Keep the solution well diluted and only consider using these products (for example, Replace and Shaklee Sport) in events lasting longer than 2 hours. If food is eaten during long training sessions or events (such as 100 km cycling), electrolytes will be provided and only water is necessary. (See appendix 9 for analysis.)

High carbohydrate drinks

Promoters of sports drinks claim these products quench thirst, provide energy and improve performance — three goals that sports participants aim to achieve. However, these drinks are generally more suitable for recovery meals.

During endurance events, between these events, or during activity that lasts all day, extra energy and delayed glycogen depletion can be provided by using a high carbohydrate drink. It is critical that these solutions are mixed correctly to control the sugar concentrations. Drinks like Gatorade (containing sucrose and glucose), Exceed (containing polycose and sucrose) and Carboplex need to be diluted to less than 10 percent carbohydrate. Consuming beverages with a higher sugar content provides no advantage and has several dis-advantages. Higher concentrations of sugar can cause blood sugar levels and hydration to be disrupted.

Glucose polymers (polycose) are often added to these drinks. Sugar solutions can cause gastric upsets because the concentration of molecules is higher in the solutions than in the body. A suitable alternative is diluted fruit juice.

High carbohydrate drinks are useful fluids for people who find it difficult to eat during events or between games.

High carbohydrate/moderate protein drinks

These are liquid meals used as part of the pre-race or pre-event meal and they should be consumed 2–3 hours before exercise. They are

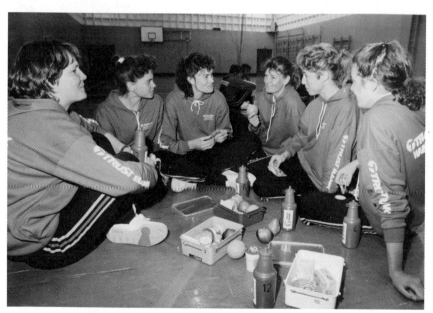

During tournaments the Waikato netball team are prepared with their snack boxes.

not considered part of fluid replacement. Examples include Ensure, Sustagen and Staminar. These drinks are useful during events only for sports participants who find it difficult to eat solid food, and only if there is sufficient time for digestion between events.

High protein drinks

Drinks high in protein are not recommended, either immediately before or during an event. These drinks are often mixed with milk, which increases the saturated fat content, further slowing down the rate of digestion. Carbohydrate is the preferred fuel during events. If using high protein formulas (Body Bulk, Protein 90), save them for after exercise, when you can replace all the energy you have burned.

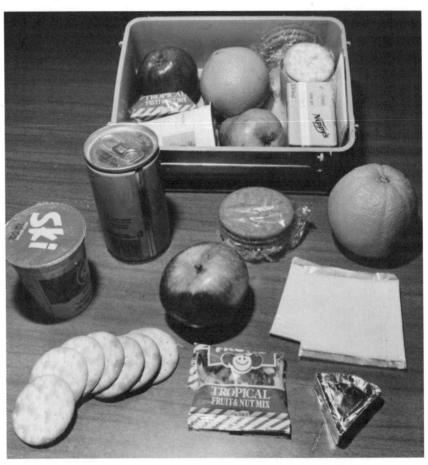

An athlete's snack box — containing high energy food to replace fuel lost during the tournament between events.

Snacks between events

Meals or foods to be eaten during competition vary depending on the game or race schedule. The most important consideration is to maintain fluid intakes. If there is more than one game or race per day the timing between each game will determine the pattern of eating. If breaks between events are long then hunger may be a problem, so eat light snacks such as crackers and fruit juice. If time between games is short, a liquid meal or fruit juices may be better. Allow sufficient time for digestion and for blood glucose levels to stabilise.

Some examples include: bananas, sandwiches or filled rolls with low fat fillings; crackers and cottage cheese or tomato; fruit purée; fruit salad; fruit juice; rice salad; and mini pizzas with tomato, a little cheese, and minimal herbs.

Endurance and ultra-endurance events

These events include the Coast-to-coast and Ironman triathlons, long distance cycling, and endurance running longer than a marathon. To maintain peak performance throughout these events, the following rules must be adhered to:

- Obtain sufficient carbohydrate for fuel.
- Eat small amounts every 15–20 minutes.
- Ensure meal breaks are well planned.
- Drink fluids regularly.

For events lasting more than one day, the meals eaten at the completion of the first day are very important (see chapter 20 for more details). Eat carbohydrate foods within the first 2 hours of completing activity.

Hyponatremia (low or reduced levels of sodium in the blood and an accompanying excess of water) has been reported in ultra-endurance running. Salt losses from sweat and consuming hypotonic solutions, which are more diluted than comparable blood concentrations, appear to be the causes. Hyponatremia is likely to afflict the average rather than the elite runner. The average runner continues running for several hours longer and drinks more hypotonic solutions. When accompanied by increased losses of salt through prolonged sweating, hyponatremia can lead to confusion, coma, seizures and oedema.

Participants in these sports must be able to judge their losses of fluid by monitoring their body weight. Weigh yourself in light underclothes before and after a 1 hour run. The environmental conditions should be as close as possible to the conditions expected for the race. Keep a record of weights and conditions for future reference. Replacement beverages should be planned and may require a combination of water and glucose electrolyte solution. During training, it is advisable to run over the ultra-endurance trail, taking food and fluids so as to assess the effectiveness and suitability of the programme.

Food for short duration activity

Some sports demand endurance or continuous activity. Others require short bursts of often intense activity or strength. The latter includes sprint events in swimming, athletics, high jump and weightlifting. In such sports there are differences in the types and groups of muscle used. The active groups of muscles may be exhausted while the inactive muscle and liver glycogen levels remain relatively unaffected.

Carbohydrate loading is not necessary for short bursts of activity and may be a disadvantage, producing muscle stiffness caused by increased water uptake by the muscle storing glycogen. The additional weight may also be a disadvantage. A moderate increase in carbohydrate foods is more sensible. A higher intake of carbohydrates a few days before the competition will increase glycogen stores and maintain blood glucose levels.

Between events, maintain adequate fluids and eat light carbohydrate snacks if events are well spaced. Remember that high intakes of sugar solutions or glucose immediately before activity will not leave the stomach in sufficient time to enter the bloodstream and this may produce some feelings of discomfort. If sugar or glucose solutions are to be used, allow enough time for blood glucose levels to stabilise before the next event.

In team events such as rugby, league, soccer, basketball and hockey, levels of activity vary greatly. The team member may be required to sprint, followed by a period of no activity, then a further sudden burst of action. The needs of each player will depend on the role or energy expenditure expected from the position played. For example, the centre position player in both hockey and netball covers a greater area than those players limited to the regions closer to the goal. Squash is another sport that is characterised by bouts of intense energy.

166

For all sports, following the baseline eating patterns and making adjustments during training to allow for energy, iron, calcium, weight control and weight maintenance will provide a solid foundation for sports performance. On the day, fine tuning is all that is required, along with additional care in maintaining fluid balance. After assessing their specific requirements and needs for their particular sport, individual sportsmen or sportswomen will be able to devise a food plan and be able to adjust their eating patterns to get peak performance from their diet.

■ ADVERSE EFFECTS OF DEHYDRATION

% of weight lost through dehydration	Symptoms
0	Normal weight
0.5–1	Thirst.
2	Stronger thirst, vague discomfort, loss of appetite.
3	Decreased performance, dry mouth, reduced urine.
4	Economy of movement.
5	Flushed skin, impatience, sleepiness, apathy, nausea, emotional instability, concentration more difficult.
6	Tingling in arms, hands, and feet; stumbling, headache, impaired temperature regulation and increase in body temperature.
8	Laboured breathing, dizziness, skin turning blue, increasing weakness, mental confusion, indistinct speech.
10	Spastic muscles, unable to balance with eyes closed, swollen tongue, delirium, general incapacity.
12	Circulatory insufficiency, concentration of blood and decreased blood volume, kidney function failing, inability to swallow.
15	Dim vision, sunken eyes, painful urination, numb skin, deafness, stiffened eyelids, cracked skin, cessation of formation of urine.
20	Barely survival limits.

(Adapted from Briggs & Galloway, *Nutrition and Physical Fitness*, W. B. Saunders Co., 1979.)

■ ■ ■

20
Recovery food

When the race or event is over, the competitors or players can regain their strength and energy by following an eating programme designed for a speedy recovery. This will enable the sports participant to refuel glycogen stores rapidly and will reduce the effects of fatigue, especially important when competition lasts for more than one day or there are several events or games in a day. There are four main nutritional areas to work on during the recovery phase. These are fluids, total energy, high carbohydrates (specifically glucose, fructose and sucrose), and the quality of the post-game meal.

Fluids

Rehydration through fluid intake should commence immediately after exercise. It can take 36–48 hours to replace fluids after a hard training session or marathon event.

Remember that thirst is not an adequate indicator of fluid needs. A light-coloured, almost clear urine indicates balanced fluid levels. A dark urine indicates concentrated levels of metabolic by-products or wastes, which means that more fluid is required because water balance has not been achieved.

Water is the best fluid. Fruit juices and sports drinks are also suitable for the recovery phase. Sports participants and athletes should be responsible for the management of their own fluids. Leave nothing to chance.

168

Carbohydrates

Glycogen depletion in muscles can occur within 2 hours of severe exercise, such as an endurance event. It can take 48 hours for muscle glycogen levels to completely recover from exercise. Some reports indicate up to 7 days may pass before glycogen is restored after an endurance event such as a marathon. The amount of glycogen in storage before exercise is relative to the length of time exercise can be performed.

When bouts of intense activity occur during the same day or over a period of days it is important to replace glycogen during the recovery phase. During continual exercise bouts, such as a netball tournament, increase carbohydrate snacks between games. Generally, baseline eating patterns, if adequate, will supply sufficient energy for performance needs, and the snacks will ward off hunger and maintain blood glucose levels.

The intake of carbohydrate after exercise increases new glycogen stores in the muscle. After exhaustive exercise it may take 24 hours before glycogen levels are completely restored, but the amount of glycogen replaced corresponds to the portion of carbohydrate eaten after exercise.

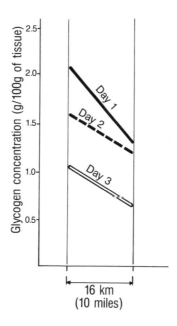

Changes in muscle glycogen levels after exeircse on 3 successive days. (Adapted from Costill et al. See Bibliography.)

As the muscles are more receptive to fuel replacement immediately after activity, carbohydrate-rich foods should be eaten within the first 2–4 hours after exercise. This will provide energy for the next day's workout. Examples of carbohydrate-rich foods are sandwiches with low fat fillings, filled rolls, pizza (wholemeal base without added cheese), pancakes, fruit juices, bananas and other fruits.

Studies have shown that consuming glucose in moderate amounts after exercise also increases glycogen replacement. Similar results have been reported with sugar. Fructose produces some increase in muscle glycogen, but the rise is less than with glucose and sugar. As fructose metabolism occurs largely in the liver, liver glycogen is increased. Very high intakes of fructose show no further increases in muscle glycogen replacement and may, in fact, induce feelings of discomfort because of the sweetness and the slowing down effect on the rate of hydration.

There appears to be no significant difference in the amount of glycogen replacement immediately after exercise, regardless of whether you use glucose and sucrose or more complex carbohydrates. However, to replace glycogen over longer periods the complex carbohydrates, or starches, appear to be the best choice.

Salt

There is no reason to take salt tablets to replace losses in sweat. Salt lost by the body will generally be replaced by the salt content of foods or salt added to the recovery meal. If salt is added remember to increase fluids as well. A lack of salt is not considered to be a problem for New Zealand sportspeople because of the amount consumed in the typical daily intake.

Potassium

After endurance exercise, additional fruits, fruit juices and vegetables that contain potassium are recommended to replace losses in sweat. Most active New Zealanders eat a wide selection of these foods in the recovery meal. Dried fruit, especially apricots, oranges, orange juice, potatoes and bananas, are excellent sources of potassium.

Fuelling the body before exercise and refuelling afterwards with adequate fluids and carbohydrates are essential for peak performance in sport. Just as no one would expect their car to run on empty, neither should the body be expected to perform on insufficient fuel. A major step towards replacing fuel is eating food immediately after workouts, training or competitive events. Recovery will be faster, more effective and the fuel source ready for the next day's training. For events lasting more than one day this procedure is crucial.

21
Eating away from home

Many races, games and events require travel. Travelling within the region, across Cook Strait or the Tasman, or to countries around the world requires special consideration because travel disrupts eating patterns. With careful planning and a little knowledge and preparation the team member or athlete can successfully overcome any problems and maintain optimum nutritional status. This will also reduce stress levels. A dramatic change in the type, amount and frequency of food eaten and changes in meal times can have serious consequences for sports performance.

Try as much as possible to continue your usual eating patterns and times established during training. However, be prepared to adapt, especially when visiting another country. It may be necessary to prepare your own meals and snacks.

In-flight and hotel meals

Check flight times and in-flight menus for international travel. Most airlines are equipped to cater for a limited number of special diets. Several are suitable for sportspeople. Arrangements should be made when booking tickets. Do not leave this until the last minute. In-flight meals are an important consideration for competitors who are required to compete within certain weight ranges. Take care with the number and type of meals eaten during long flights. It is very easy to consume more food than normal because of boredom or the stress of flying long distances. Water is the best fluid. Dilute fruit juices with

172

water or soda water, or use plenty of ice. As strong tea, coffee and large volumes of cola beverages act as diuretics, disrupting fluid balance, keep these to a minimum or well diluted. If fresh water is unavailable or the safety of local water supply is suspect, choose bottled water or bottled beverages that are low in sugar.

Alcohol contributes to fatigue and dehydration as well as impairing coordination and performance. The consumption of alcohol during air travel is best avoided, especially before an event. Save it until the trip home, but remember it will delay the recovery phase.

Keep meals light and high in carbohydrate. Eat fresh fruit, fruit salads, cereals and plenty of vegetables. Watch out for temptations that are high in fat, such as rich cakes, fried foods, batters and pastry. Avoid foods containing large amounts of butter, oil, cheese, cream and chocolate. Takeaway foods should be selected with care. It is possible to choose a takeaway meal that meets nutritional requirements and is not hazardous to performance.

Try not to add salt to foods and avoid foods that are high in salt. In countries with hot or tropical climates salt requirements are slightly higher, but a little added to the meal is all that is required.

Watch snacks. Choose high quality carbohydrate-based snacks and limit or avoid snacks that are high in fat, sugar or salt. These can be replaced with sandwiches, fresh fruit, fruit juices, fat-reduced

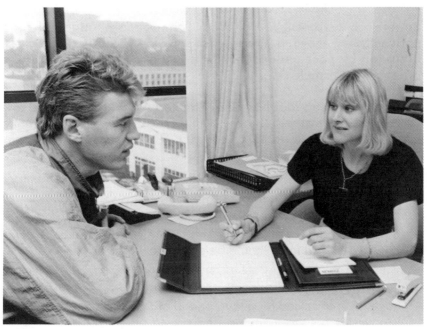

John Kirwan discusses his nutritional requirements with the author.

173

yoghurts, plain muesli bars and dried fruit. Always carry some of your own snacks, but beware of customs regulations when travelling overseas as certain food items may be confiscated for agricultural reasons.

Maintain weight. Monitor weight loss or gain caused by stress or the unlimited availability of food. Some sportspeople find their appetite is reduced or increased during periods of rest or travel.

Hotel accommodation can be a trap for the inexperienced. Coaches and administrators must be aware of the types of food served at hotels in countries where the food is different from that which the players are accustomed to. Phoning ahead and organising meals avoids the frustrations of not being able to identify food items on the menu or finding meals unsuitable, and will also relieve stress. These preparations all help smooth the journey.

Eat foods that are familiar. Save the more adventurous items and new foods until after the event. Experiment on the way home, when there will be no effect on performance. Before the event, stick to what you know and enjoy.

Food poisoning

Beware of the possibility of food poisoning. An attack of food poisoning will leave a sportsperson weak, dehydrated, fatigued, frustrated by poor performance or even unable to compete. There are some very simple steps to follow:

- Never eat food that has been handled many times. Ensure raw food is well washed. Choose whole foods where possible. Make sure food is fresh and kept covered. Do not eat food that looks or smells strange.

- Check that water is drinkable. If unsure, boil it first. Remember that ice in drinks is also made from the local water.

- Test the temperature of the foods when served. Hot food should be served hot, not lukewarm. This is particularly relevant to pies and stews. Cold food should be completely cold.

- Take special care with seafood, especially if the location of the event is a long way from the sea. Selecting seafood dishes that have been unchilled for a long period of time is asking for trouble. Watch out for those shrimp and prawn filled rolls left sitting in the sun or on the servery or display for a few hours.

- Never reheat food, and do not keep meat, egg or dairy-based dishes warm for long periods of time.

Fortunately, the use of the microwave has helped, as foods can now be heated straight from the refrigerator, rather than being kept in a warming oven for long periods.

If you are unfortunate enough to contract food poisoning consult the team doctor immediately. Sip diluted fluids as much as possible to maintain fluid balance and begin by eating low fibre foods until fully recovered.

Food in a foreign country

When eating in a foreign country, special precautions must be taken before a sports event.

- Take care with unfamiliar food and food served out of doors.

- Watch spices. New Zealanders' digestive systems are generally not equipped to handle the highly spiced foods served in some countries.

- Ask for sauces, dressings and gravy to be served separately so you can decide the amount to be added. In some countries large servings of oil-based dressings or mayonnaise are added to salads before service.

- Choose meals such as grilled fish or chicken with wholemeal bread, potato or pasta. Salad rolls with light fillings are an excellent choice for lunches. Remember to keep up the carbohydrate content of the meals.

- Watch the sauces added to pasta meals. Some of these are high in oil, fat and cheese which increases the fat content of the meal. Take care with the amount of spices and garlic used.

- If the meal contains more salt than you are used to, increase your fluids. Drink more water or fruit juice with the meal.

- When dining out at restaurants don't be afraid to ask what is in a dish if it appears unrecognisable. It is then possible to work out how the dish fits into the basic guidelines for good nutrition.

- Aim for variety and save special treat foods until after the event.

Dining out

The most popular takeaway meals are fish and chips, fried chicken and hamburgers. Convenience foods are also fast foods. They are easy to prepare and often require the addition of one simple ingredient and fresh vegetables or fruit to complement the meal. For the athlete, getting maximum nutrition for the dollar can be a concern.

During training or when travelling to events there are many opportunities to dine out. This can break the monotony of travel or a training programme without being hazardous to performance. However, remember that takeaways and dining out are not intended to provide a complete diet but to provide one meal as part of an overall eating pattern. There is no need to avoid takeaways or dining out with friends in their home or at a restaurant, provided a few general guidelines are followed.

Restaurant food

Check ahead first. Ask the receptionist or head waiter to describe a selection of the dishes on the menu. Provided sufficient warning is given, many chefs are happy to provide a suitable alternative or perhaps a special request. Build up a good line of communication with individual restaurants and future service and cooperation will become easier. Many restaurants are familiar with the Pritikin style of cooking and the recent efforts of the Heart Foundation have heightened awareness of the role of food and sound nutrition. Be prepared to ask what is in a dish and the size of servings.

If you are dining out in another country, ask the local administrators for recommendations of suitable places to eat, and make sure you provide them with sufficient information about the style and type of food preferred. But remember that it is the individual's responsibility to attend to his or her own meals.

The following guidelines should be applied to restaurant dining:

- Select dishes that are grilled, baked, steamed or lightly poached. Foods cooked in fat, oil or surrounded with pastry are not recommended.

- Ask for all sauces to be served separately or on the side. This includes rich creamy sauces as well as gravy and dressings.

- Select fruit juices and ask for a jug of iced water with the meal.

- Dishes that are heavily spiced or salted should be avoided.

- Choose potatoes baked or microwaved in their jackets rather than fried, chipped or roasted.

- Select wholegrain breads, rolls, plain biscuits or crackers and use only a small amount of butter or margarine.

- To bulk up meals, request additional servings of rice, pasta (preferably wholegrain) or potatoes and other vegetables. Ensure that they do not contain added fat, butter, margarine, oil or sauces.

- Select fresh fruit, fruit salads, fruit sorbets or light fruit-based desserts. Fat-reduced yoghurt is recommended to replace ice cream and heavy, rich sauces.

- If alcohol is included, the choice of drink is important. Limit the amount and number of alcoholic drinks to one or two servings. Dilute wine with soda water and/or ice. Choose low alcohol beers and use low calorie mixers, such as soda water, or sugar-free lemonade, cordials or cola, with spirits.

Takeaways

Takeaways are not necessarily junk food. Some sound nutritional decisions can make all the difference, making takeaway food a sensible alternative for a quick meal. Although not recommended as a regular part of the diet, fast foods or takeaways provide variety and convenience when included occasionally in the meal pattern.

Fast foods as an occasional treat cause no significant damage to health and performance. However, people who regularly eat out at takeaway outlets more than two to three times a week have cause for concern.

Some fast foods, because of the method of cooking and the nature of the food, are high in saturated fat, energy, salt and sugar and low in vitamins A and C, iron, calcium and complex carbohydrates, especially fibre. It is the percentage of energy supplied from fat that causes problems for the sportsperson. Some meals provide 45–50 percent of the energy as fat. *Nutritional Recommendations for New Zealanders* advises a decrease to below 30 percent, so a high fat meal limits the fat intake for the rest of the day. In addition, the fat in takeaway meals is generally saturated, which contributes to raised cholesterol levels in the blood. When considering the energy content of fast foods remember that these foods are a meal, not a snack.

Unless fresh fruit or salad are included, fast foods tend to be low in vitamins, particularly vitamin C. Heat-sensitive vitamins are destroyed when held for a long time at high temperatures. As well as vitamin C, thiamine (vitamin B_1) is also at risk. A hamburger can provide significant intakes of protein, iron and zinc, and the inclusion of dairy products (cheese or milk) will increase the calcium intake.

High intakes of sugar can occur through additional items ordered with the main meal. Foods such as sweet soda drinks, milkshakes, thickshakes, sundaes, ice cream and other desserts contain high sugar levels. Choosing low fat milks, fruit juice, soda water or even plain water will keep sugar intake at an acceptable level. Fast foods that are high in fibre include tacos, corn chips and wholemeal pizzas.

Fish and chips   Request that no salt be added and leave the tomato sauce and tartare sauce behind. Use lemon juice or vinegar instead. Serve a fresh salad, or at least fresh fruits, with the meal. Remove the batter from the fish and do not add extra salt. One large piece of fish in batter (1 680 kJ) with a scoop of chips (1 386 kJ) totals 3 066 kJ (730 Cal)! Take note of how frequently fish and chips appears on the monthly or weekly menu. If turning up regularly select the battered fish on one occasion and the chips the next, adding your own vegetables or fish. Add a carton of low fat milk to the meal to improve calcium intake.

Hamburgers   Wholemeal buns and lean fillings will help to improve the standard hamburger. Request additional salad where possible and ask for no added salt. Order a small serving of chips or replace these with fruit. Select fresh fruit, fruit juice and milk rather than sweet soda beverages. Watch for the extras of double cheese, double meat, egg, and bacon and cheese, which increase the salt and fat intake. Where possible, ask for a grilled bun and meat, rather than fried. Home-made hamburgers make an excellent meal and are quick, economical and easy to prepare.

Fried chicken   Removing the skin and any batter will lower the fat content significantly. Barbecued and rotisseried chicken are the preferred choices. Instead of chips, select vegetables (coleslaw, corn cob, potato salad, bean salad) and bread rolls. Add a carton of low fat milk, or fresh fruit or fruit juice to finish the meal.

Pizza   Try not to make a meal out of pizza alone. Select the small and average sizes to reduce overeating. Add salads, fresh fruit, fruit juice, and low fat milk. Watch the high fat and high salt toppings. These include double cheese, anchovies, ham, tuna, bacon bits, seafoods, olives and salami. Include more toppings such as green peppers, mushrooms, tomato, onion and pineapple.

Chinese   Ask for monosodium glutamate (MSG) and soya sauce to be excluded. Choose meals that are mostly vegetables, such as chop suey, chow mein and rice dishes. Request steamed rice and noodles rather than the fried selection. Keep deep-fried foods, lemon sauces and sweet-and-sour sauces for a special occasion. Chinese food uses only small amounts of meat, usually fish, beef, chicken or pork. Check the meat portion is not battered and deep-fried before being included in the dish; meat for sweet-and-sour dishes is usually prepared this way. Add low fat milk to complement the meal.

Pies and sausage rolls These foods are very high in fat — one pie contains over five teaspoons. Many active people can easily consume two meat pies for lunch. Some people can eat this for morning tea, particularly if they have missed beakfast. Ten teaspoons of fat equals 1 900 kJ (over 450 Cal) without considering the flour and filling. An occasional pie does no harm, but include a salad, salad sandwich, fresh fruit, fruit juice or fat-reduced milk with the pie or sausage roll to provide less fat and salt, more fibre, vitamins and calcium. If pies are kept warm for long periods many of the B vitamins are destroyed as they are sensitive to heat.

■ *RATING TAKEAWAYS PER AVERAGE SERVING*

Food	Energy	Fat	CHO	Pro-tein	Salt	Fibre	Rating
Fish & chips	3 066	***	***	***	***	*	1
Burger (McD)	946	*	**	**	*	*	3
Burger (other)	1 273	**	**	**	**	*	2
Fried chicken	2 469	***	***	***	***	*	1
Chinese chicken	3 289	*	***	***	***	***	3
Pie & sandwich	2 355	***	**	**	**	*	2
Pizza	3 543	**	***	***	***	***	2
Wholegrain sandwich & carrot cake & fruit	3 578	**	***	***	**	***	4

Code: * low, ** moderate, *** high
Overall rating: 1 (poor) to 4 (good)

■ ■ ■

Recommended takeaway meals include:

Wholegrain salad rolls or salad sandwiches.
Sandwiches, fruit and low fat milk.
Fruit salad, fruit juice and reduced fat milk.

Fresh fruit, rice salad and coleslaw.
Grilled chicken and lean meat with salad or vegetables.
Spaghetti or pasta with savoury tomato sauce.
Beans, bean salad and vegetables.
Frozen meals without pastry and fresh vegetables.
Pre-cooked chicken without batter or skin, and salad.
Stir-fry Chinese meals (chop suey, chow mein) and fresh fruit.
Hamburger and salad, with fruit juice and fresh fruit.
Pizza with salad and fruit.

22
Reading food labels

When training schedules leave little time available for shopping, sports people tend to rely on convenience foods. It is important, therefore, to select the maximum nutritional value for your dollar. Convenience foods are quick to prepare but need to be chosen with care. More attention is now being placed on the quality of food, in terms of nutrition and safety. Food labels assist the athlete to identify the ingredients that go into a product, list certain food additives included during manufacture, and protect the purchaser from unscrupulous operators.

By reading the ingredient labels on products you will be able to compare different foods in terms of salt content per serving, energy supplied by fat, fibre content, and levels of simple carbohydrates (sugar and glucose).

Most packaged food labels are required to list, in descending order (by weight), all the ingredients contained in the food. If fat is listed among the first two or three ingredients the product will be high in fat. Look for unsaturated fat, though many manufacturers are using the statement 'contains animal or vegetable fat', which makes it difficult to identify which fat has actually been used. An additive is currently listed by its function rather than the name of the additive used; for example, 'preservative', 'colour', 'stabiliser', 'flavour' or 'emulsifier'.

By reading the labels, different brands or varieties of a food can be compared and the lower fat (saturated and unsaturated), lower salt and higher fibre qualities can be identified. Quantities are often listed per serving or per 100 g.

181

Information found on a packaged food product varies considerably depending largely on the individual manufacturer. Some or all of the following details may be present.

Name and address   The name and address of the manufacturer or importer must be clearly identified. A postal address is not sufficient.

Barcode   Many supermarkets now use electronic scanners to record the price and product. The number also identifies the country of origin, the manufacturing company and the name of the individual product.

Instructions for storage   The manufacturer will often provide instructions for the storage of the product, to maintain the best possible quality.

Net weight   This describes the actual weight of the food at processing, excluding the package and wrapping.

Use-by date   Perishable products should have a use-by date. This indicates the time the food remains at the best quality. Although the food does not deteriorate or spoil immediately after that date it is possible its quality has declined. Some products may carry a date that indicates when the product was manufactured. This is usually written as 'Packed on . . . '

Country of origin   Imported products often display the country of origin — for example, 'Product of Australia' or 'Product of Denmark'. Some New Zealand-made items are appearing with a symbol and the statement 'Product of NZ'.

Nutrition labelling   Information provided here varies considerably, from the number of calories or kilojoules per unit serving (or per 100 g) to a more detailed analysis of the composition of the product. The number of kilojoules may be listed as per serving or as a percentage of the energy value of the food. The different types of fat (saturated or unsaturated) and cholesterol content may also be listed. Information such as 'no added sugar', 'no added salt' or 'sweetened with fruit juice' may appear. This information is useful for those interested in weight control and for diabetics.

Ingredient listing   All ingredients are listed in descending order by weight, the largest ingredient listed first. If the nutritional content label is absent, this list provides a useful guide to the composition of the product. If honey, sugar, glucose, butter, margarine or oil are listed in the first few ingredients it is likely the product is high in energy. Additives also appear in this list.

When selecting food based on food labels the important points to identify are:

- serving size;
- percentage and type of fat;
- added or hidden sugar;
- added or hidden salt — look for 'no added salt' on label;
- the cost of the convenience food, compared to do-it-yourself preparation;
- marketing terms, such as lite, light, lean and health food — these terms may be advertising only and do not necessarily imply health benefits.

Nutrient content

Nutrient labelling tells you the nutrients contained in each serving. The carbohydrate content refers to all the various types of carbohydrates and includes complex carbohydrate (flour, oats, rice, coconut, nuts) and simple carbohydrates (fruit juice, honey, malt, sugar, fructose, glucose and the sugar provided by fruits). The different types of carbohydrates and sugars are often listed separately, so as to appear less prominent on the label. Dietary fibre may or may not be listed independently.

Sodium quantities indicate the amount of salt (sodium chloride) present. On many products this is not listed. Some product labels may state 'no salt added'.

Calorie content can be listed as energy value or calories or kilojoules per unit, serving or 100 g. Vitamins and minerals are sometimes listed and this provides useful information for people interested in specific nutrients, for example iron and calcium.

Food additives

There is an increasing demand by consumers to limit or reduce the number of preservatives and additives in foods. Some products now appear with the statement 'contains no preservatives, no artificial flavouring or colourings'. Other additives are often used to enhance the keeping qualities of the product, such as emulsifiers, which stop ingredients from separating.

183

Some people are allergic or sensitive to certain substances. Food labels help to identify food containing these substances so that those who are allergic can avoid them and choose a similar food without the additive.

In the next 2–3 years a new system that will give more information on food labels is to be phased in. The specific name of an additive, or its code number, will be listed. Foods imported from England and Europe use the same numbering system that will be used in New Zealand, except that each additive on an English product is prefixed with the letter 'E'. Australia also lists food additives on some products. Each approved additive has its own number, which means that long scientific names can be easily coded. Additives that do not have code numbers will be identified by name. (For a list of permitted additives and their codes, see appendix 7.)

Food additives have allowed a dramatic increase in the number and variety of foods available. Without food additives many foods would not be available or would be unattractive in terms of colour and flavour.

Some of the additives used in food processing today have been used for many years, even centuries. These include common foods such as sugar, salt, spices, smoke for preserving, and vinegar. Some of these are found naturally in foods.

Additives are included in manufactured food for a number of reasons: to improve its appearance, flavour, colour or consistency; to maintain nutritional quality; and to enhance its keeping quality or stability.

Some common food additives and their functions are:

Colour   Added to replace colour lost during processing, to enhance natural colour, or to create unique colours. Colour is added to reinforce flavour.

Flavour and flavour enhancers   Can be natural or synthetic; they provide a standard product or are used to enhance food flavours.

Preservatives   Control the growth of undesirable bacteria, mould and yeasts which cause 'off' flavours, texture changes and deterioration.

Antioxidant   Minimises changes due to oxygen and is used in foods containing fats and oils. Oxidation can produce an unpleasant flavour and colour changes in these substances.

Enzymes   Prevent cloudiness in beer and tenderise meat; also used to make cheese and yoghurt from milk.

184

Emulsifiers and thickeners Modify textures, thicken foods, and stabilise oil and vinegar mixtures.

Food acids Provide consistent levels of acid in food.

Flour treatment agents Make flour more suitable for baking.

Anti-caking agent Added to finely powdered foods such as salt or sugar to prevent clumping and to allow product to flow freely when poured.

Moisturising agents or humectants Prevent products drying out and help maintain a soft texture in some foods.

Phosphates Enhance texture of processed meats.

Propellants Used to propel food from pressurised or aerosol food containers.

Artificial sweeteners Substances with intense sweetness, used in small quantities to sweeten foods.

23
Nutritional concerns for sportswomen

Women have many demands placed on their health during a lifetime. The first major increase in nutritional requirements comes with the growth spurt and onset of menstruation in adolescence. Pregnancy and lactation (breastfeeding) also impose high nutritional demands, as do the changes associated with menopause. The food eaten throughout her life plays an important role in health and sports performance for the active woman. Obtaining an adequate intake of energy and iron appear to be the most difficult nutritional tasks.

When comparing the average male with the average female some differences are evident. The average female is 8–10 cm shorter, 11–13 kg lighter, and has 4.5–7 kg more fat tissue and 18–20 kg less lean tissue (including muscle, bone and organs) than the average man.

Women can gain a number of health benefits through participation in sport. With moderate intensity training programmes, significant decreases in blood cholesterol and blood pressure, decreased body fat, and increased lean tissue have been reported. It appears that women athletes are generally more positive about themselves and their bodies than non-athletic women. However, lower iron levels have also been reported in sportswomen, which is not beneficial.

186

Baseline eating patterns

The sportswoman should follow the same basic principles for optimum nutrition as the sportsman. Maintaining a regular pattern of eating will prevent the development of nutrient deficiencies. By adhering to the guidelines from the basic foods groups and selecting foods from each group daily, a balanced intake of nutrients can be achieved. The following are some suggested foods from each of the four groups, which are suitable for the sportswoman's daily menu.

Milk group
Minimum number of servings = 2
1 cup low fat milk or fat reduced yoghurt, 40 g cheese, 2 cups cottage cheese or ice cream.
Many women have eliminated milk from the food plan thinking it will assist with weight reduction. This severely reduces one of the best sources of calcium.

Meat group
Minimum number of servings = 2
50-75 g lean meat, chicken or fish, 2 eggs, 50 g cheese, 1 cup dried legumes.
It is important to choose lean or low fat sources of protein and to pay particular attention to those food sources that are excellent sources of iron.

Fruit/vegetable group
Minimum number of servings = 4
½ cup juice, ½ cup cooked vegetables or fruit, 1 cup raw vegetable or fruit, ½ grapefruit, ¼ melon.
Fruits and vegetables provide valuable sources of vitamins, fibre and water, and add variety to the food plan. Take care not to add sugar or salt. Fruit and vegetables are better eaten raw, or with only the minimal amount of cooking.

Cereals/grain group
Minimum number of servings = 4
1 slice bread, preferably wholegrain, 30 g cereal, ½ cup cooked cereal (porridge), ½ cup pasta, ½ cup rice, ½ cup muesli.
Cereals and grains are excellent sources of fibre and B vitamins, and provide bulk in the food plan. Wholegrain cereals can also provide some additional iron.

By eating the recommended number of servings from each food group it is possible to obtain all the nutrients necessary for good health.

187

Sportswomen and other active individuals will also need to increase the servings of fruits, vegetables, cereals and grains to provide added carbohydrate for activity. Remember, these are the minimum servings. Every woman is an individual and adjustment should be made accordingly.

Some additional health concerns for women are: weight control and weight maintenance, osteoporosis, premenstrual syndrome and iron deficiency. Special attention must also be given to the growth phases of adolescence, pregnancy and lactation.

Weight concerns

Many women feel concern about weight and body shape. The percentage of women who feel they are overweight appears higher among elite female athletes. Some sportswomen believe a thinner, lighter body will provide a competitive advantage. However, no relationship has been shown between a lighter body weight and faster times. Most sportswomen are aware that being overweight means using more energy to move and is less energy efficient, but the opposite (an underweight body has more energy, resulting in faster times) is not valid. In fact, extremely low body fat and body weights can be detrimental to performance.

Weight loss and weight gain require equal attention. Sportswomen must still obtain adequate energy for training while they are on a weight loss programme. Fad diets, high protein drinks or missing meals compromises sports performance. A realistic goal must be established.

For weight gain, more nutrient-dense food and snacks that provide an additional 2.1 MJ per day will increase weight by around 500g per week. It is important that exercise continues, so as to avoid an increase in fat weight. (For further details refer to chapter 12.) Thinness in women appears to increase the risk of developing osteoporosis, and excess weight does seem to offer some protection against this disease.

Sports such as gymnastics, figure skating, long distance running, dancing and bodybuilding require a low body weight and body fat level. Some of these sportswomen may be consuming less energy than expected because of their adaptation to exercise. This improved ability to exercise on lower energy levels may explain why some women eat very little and maintain activity levels. Very low energy diets are not recommended for sportswomen.

There is also a higher prevalence of reported eating disorders (such as anorexia and bulimia) among elite athletes. Reports also indicate that these women restrict food choices and limit red meat, sugar, salt, processed foods and ice cream. It is important that sportswomen establish realistic weight goals and body fat percentages relative to their particular sport. This is often a matter of education. Eating disorders require special attention as such behaviour can result in wide swings in weight, mood and performance. Establishing realistic eating patterns is essential and needs the help of a supportive team made up of the coach, doctor and dietitian.

Calcium and osteoporosis

A nutritionally adequate food intake and regular exercise play an important role in the development and maintenance of bone and the skeleton. New Zealand has one of the highest incidences of osteoporosis in the world. One out of every four women over the age of 60 develops osteoporosis. One woman in three suffers from a fracture as a result of osteoporosis. Fractures usually involve the wrist, hip or spine. Each year about 2 000 New Zealand women break a hip.

Women are more prone to osteoporosis than men because of their smaller skeletal frame and the period of bone loss that occurs following menopause. Women tend to lose twice the calcium lost by men. Changes in female hormones which occur around menopause result in an accelerated loss of calcium from the bones. Thin women, women with low body fat levels, and elite athletes whose high exercise intensities cause menstruation to stop are more prone to this problem. There is some concern that low intakes of protein in these women are an additional factor.

Although researchers are as yet unable to show a direct relationship between dietary calcium intake and the incidence of osteoporosis, insufficient calcium in the diet is considered to be a contributing factor. Several studies indicate a relationship between the consumption of calcium during the teenage years and the amount of bone mass in later years. Consumption of milk and other dairy products during childhood can be important for future bone density. Obtaining adequate calcium begins in early adolescence and continues throughout life.

Moderate exercise helps prevent osteoporosis, but heavy training can have the opposite effect. Weight-bearing exercise (walking, carrying objects, climbing stairs) appears to have a beneficial effect. However, our modern lifestyle has reduced the amount of this activity. Limiting food intake, as in strict dieting or eating disorders (bulimia, anorexia nervosa), and reducing or eliminating dairy foods from eating patterns further aggravates this problem. Keeping body fat at suitable levels for normal menstruation and maintaining adequate calcium and protein intakes are particularly important for young sportswomen.

Tips for maintaining calcium intake

- As exercise plays a role in calcium metabolism, keep active, not just during the season, but throughout the year. Use the stairs instead of the lift.

- If participating in heavy training take extra care to include calcium-rich food sources regularly in meals.

- Get enough sunlight for vitamin D production, as this vitamin assists with the absorption of calcium. About half an hour a day appears sufficient.

- Take a reasonable amount of calcium regularly throughout life. Female hormones affect bones at different times during the lifespan. During menopause changes in hormone levels increase calcium loss from bone. The earlier in life that adequate calcium is included in the usual eating pattern the more benefit is provided in the long term.

- If you dislike milk, use cheese sauces for vegetables, grated cheese on salads, tofu and other soya bean products, custards, rice puddings, macaroni cheese, and yoghurt on porridge and cereals, for lunch, or as a yoghurt shake for a snack.

- Eat tinned fish (salmon, sardines) regularly.

- Eat dark-green-leaf vegetables regularly, fresh or raw if possible. Oranges and broccoli also contain calcium. Some foods (sesame

■ FOODS RATED ACCORDING TO CALCIUM CONTENT

Rich	Medium	Poor
Milk	Whole cereals	Egg
Cheese	Green veg	Fruit
Cottage cheese	Beans	Butter and margarine
Yoghurt	Nuts	Fats and oils
Ice cream		Cream
Chocolate		Refined cereals
Custard		Potato
Salmon		Rice (white)
Shrimps		Pasta
Tofu		

■ ■ ■

190

seeds, spinach, silverbeet, celery leaves, rhubarb) contain chemicals, called phytates and oxalates, that bind calcium, making it unavailable for absorption. However, it is unlikely that these foods influence the calcium in other foods eaten at the same meal.

● Excessive quantities of protein are not recommended as high intakes of protein reduce the amount of calcium absorbed. Increasing the protein from 50 to 100 g will halve the absorption of calcium. Further calcium losses occur with a high salt intake.

● Caffeine, from cola drinks, tea, coffee and chocolate, interferes with the absorption of calcium. Keep alcohol intake to a minimum

■ CALCIUM CONTENT OF CERTAIN FOODS

Food	Serving	Calcium mg
Trim milk	200 ml	320
Cheese: gruyère	25 g (1 slice)	294
Sesame seeds	1 tbsp (25 g)	291
2-Ten milk	200 ml	280
Yoghurt	200 g	250
Whole milk	200 ml	240
Swiss cheese	25 g (1 slice)	240
Salmon	100 g	190
Cheddar cheese	25 g (1 slice)	200
Sardines	50 g (4 large)	187
Processed cheese	25 g (1 slice)	160
Milk chocolate	50 g	150
Cottage cheese	125 g	120
Parmesan cheese	1 tsp (10 g)	120
Almonds	50 g ($^1/3$ cup)	120
Tofu	100 g	120
Broccoli	100 g	100
Silverbeet/puha	½ cup cooked	65
Kidney/baked beans	½ cup (115 g)	50
Orange	1	55
Bread: white/grain	3 slices	35
Dried apricots	5 (30 g)	30
Egg	1 (50 g)	25
Rolled oats	½ cup cooked	15
Kumara	½ cup	15
Pumpkin	½ cup	15
Meat/chicken	150 g serving	15
Potato	100 g (1 baked)	10

■ ■ ■

and avoid smoking as both alcohol and nicotine reduce calcium absorption.

- The calcium from calcium supplements is not as well absorbed as the calcium in foods such as milk. Take care not to exceed recommended doses. In some people excess calcium may lead to kidney stones because their hormones do not control calcium absorption properly.

- Eat a wide variety of foods and include servings of calcium-rich foods regularly.

Consuming calcium-rich foods is the best way to meet daily calcium requirements. If taking supplements, use small doses to complement dietary intake. High doses of calcium through supplements is causing some concern among scientists because it has been found to alter absorption of iron and zinc. (For further information, see discussion on calcium in chapter 10.)

Premenstrual tension

Before menstruation begins many women feel tired, restless, hungry, depressed or moody. Some experience cravings for sweet or salty foods; others feel bloated or gain weight. Some may experience tender or swollen breasts. One or more of these symptoms can be experienced during the week, or a few days, before periods begin.

Hormone changes in the menstrual cycle are associated with PMT (premenstrual tension). Salt or sodium balance may also be affected. Some treatments prescribed for PMT, such as large doses of vitamins or hormones, are ineffective and can be unsafe. Large doses of vitamin B_6 are often used in the belief that this will relieve mood changes, but, to date, no studies have supported a definite benefit. Evening primrose oil, an oil rich in fatty acids, was also thought to relieve the symptoms because it was thought that PMT was caused by a fatty acid deficiency. However, present research has failed to show fatty acid deficiencies in women with PMT.

A few changes can be made to a balanced food plan, which may help to relieve PMT symptoms:

- Drink more water. Reducing the caffeine may help if breasts are swollen and tender, so limit the use of coffee (other than decaffeinated), tea, cola drinks and chocolate.

- Eat more frequently to reduce feelings of hunger and food cravings. Spread the usual food intake over five to six meals during the day, but try not to eat additional food.

- Eat less salty foods and avoid adding salt to food at the table. Reducing salt intake may help reduce water retention and the consequent bloated feeling.

- Some weight gain is normal just before or during your period so stay away from the scales; it only makes you more depressed if you are trying to reduce weight at this time.

- Taking light or moderate exercise can help. Try a walk, light jog, swim or cycle for fun, but avoid turning it into a training session.

- Limit the use of alcohol. Research has reported that alcohol has a more intoxicating effect on many women just before the onset and in the first few days of the period.

- Eat a wide variety of foods, especially fruits and vegetables.

These techniques may help some sportswomen. There is no guarantee they will work for everyone. See your doctor if your PMT symptoms are severe.

Iron deficiency

(For a full discussion, see chapter 10.)

Iron is a special concern for women, particularly women athletes. Lifecycle changes (growth spurts, pregnancy and lactation) increase the demand for iron, in addition to regular monthly losses through menstruation. Women who experience heavy menstrual periods, have had several pregnancies, or use an intra-uterine device (IUD) should check for iron deficiency.

Very restrictive slimming diets fail to provide adequate iron. Many women who eliminate meat from their eating patterns in an attempt to cut kilojoules remove one of the best sources of iron.

If sportswomen express feelings of tiredness, training fails to show the improvement expected, or performance is reduced, iron levels and energy intakes need to be assessed. A low intake of iron is a common nutritional problem for women throughout the world, and iron deficiency significantly compromises sports performance.

193

The following guidelines will help you to get enough iron in your diet:

- Include a wide variety of rich sources of iron in the food plan. These include lean meats, liver, chicken, lamb, veal, pork, venison and fish.

- Choose wholegrain cereals and breads.

- Include a rich source of vitamin C with meals as this enhances the absorption of iron.

- Drink tea, coffee and cola beverages in moderation as these drinks can reduce the amount of iron the body absorbs.

- If regularly competing in endurance events, monitor your iron status (haemoglobin and ferritin levels).

- Iron is absorbed best from foods. Supplements may be used to correct a deficiency but long-term food choices need to be improved.

Teenage sportswomen

During their teenage years sportswomen undergo a number of body changes that place additional demands on their nutritional requirements. The growth spurt demands additional energy and increases in all nutrients. The onset of menstruation increases the requirement for iron.

The young sportswoman requires more protein (2-3 g extra per day depending on training), iron, calcium, phosphorus and vitamin B than adults. Energy levels increase to over 8.4 MJ per day. This varies, however, according to training and the individual energy expenditure of each sport. These energy demands are required for the tremendous growth in lean tissue and bone, and for the increased fat weight before the onset of menstruation.

Menstruation begins significantly later in sportswomen than in their non-exercising counterparts. This is probably related to the type of sport and the level of competition. For most women, menstruation appears to have no effect on sports performance. Consequently, young sportswomen should be allowed to train and compete in sporting activities during menstruation, provided they are comfortable and are suffering no unpleasant symptoms which could affect performance.

194

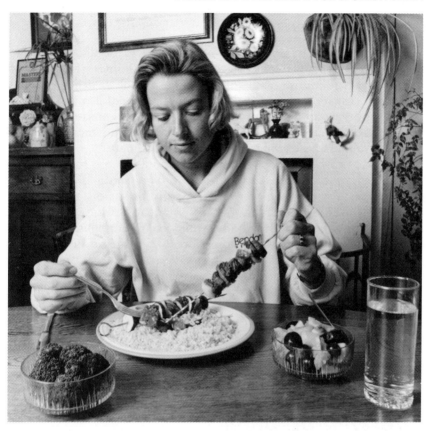

New Zealand netball star Sandra Edge (Mallett) combines an intake of lean red meat with vitamin C-rich fresh fruit salad to increase her absorption of iron.

■ ENERGY EXPENDITURE DURING EXERCISE BY A 55 KG WOMAN

Light exercise (8–16 kJ/min)	Moderate (16–24 kJ/min)	High (24+ kJ/min)
archery	badminton	athletics
bowls	canoeing	basketball
cricket	cycling	climbing
golf	gymnastics	cross country
sailing	hockey	soccer
table tennis	jogging	rowing
volleyball	swimming	squash
	tennis	
	walking	

■ ■ ■

Amenorrhoea

Mild to moderate exercise does not appear to significantly affect menstruation or result in any related disorders. Of interest is the lower incidence of painful periods (or dysmenorrhoea) in active women. However, cessation of menstruation (amenorrhoea) has been found in some sportswomen performing heavy intensive exercise or training. This appears more common in ballet dancers and marathon and distance runners. In addition to high exercise intensity, other factors that appear to be associated with this condition are low body fat percentages and previous irregularities with menstruation. Low levels of hormones and protein in the diet may also be factors.

Amenorrhoea appears to be a temporary state and normal menstruation occurs once the heavy training is discontinued. The main concern for sportswomen with amenorrhoea is increasing evidence showing that this can increase the possibility of developing osteoporosis, in a similar way to that of post-menopausal women. There also appears to be a higher incidence of stress fractures among women with amenorrhoea. Calcium may be low and, in some cases, medical advice may involve the inclusion of a calcium supplement for these women.

By consuming a diet that provides adequate iron, calcium and energy, sportswomen of a healthy weight may prevent amenorrhea.

Oral contraception

Nutritional status may be altered through the use of the oral contraceptive pill. It is not known if there is any detrimental effect to performance caused by oral contraceptives, but there is an indication that certain vitamins and minerals may require special attention, particularly folate and vitamin B_6. Women taking oral contraceptives appear to have higher levels of vitamin A in the blood, so vitamin A supplements are not recommended.

Pregnancy and lactation

Complications in pregnancy and childbirth are fewer in sportswomen than in non-exercising females. Childbirth does not adversely affect sporting performance. This will return to normal levels within 1–2 years, depending on training.

There are, however, several additional demands placed on nutrient intakes during pregnancy and breastfeeding. There is a general need to increase all nutrients, but in particular iron (because of the increase in blood volume during the development of the foetus), folate and calcium for bone development. Often pregnant women are prescribed an iron folate supplement, and occasionally calcium.

Weight training

Changes in body composition resulting from weight training are similar to those that occur with increased training. There is a noticeable decrease in body fat (around 2.5–3 kg), a smaller increase in lean tissue (muscle) and a small decrease in total body weight. This depends on the initial body composition of the sportswoman before training. Therefore, these changes will be less pronounced in lean athletes than overweight or obese individuals. Dietary modification must also be involved to provide a sensible weight loss programme without affecting lean muscle mass or performance.

During the off-season, or at the end of a sporting career, if some form of moderate exercise is not maintained and eating habits adjusted, almost all of the changes that occurred during training will be reversed.

Post-menopause

There are many sportswomen who remain active through the later years of their life; some will compete at the World Veteran Games. With the decrease in basal metabolism that occurs with age, there may be a corresponding increase in weight. However, the major nutrition-related problem is osteoporosis. It appears that exercise can have a beneficial effect and delay any further thinning of the bone. In some cases oestrogen (female hormone) replacement may be necessary to prevent or halt this condition.

More calcium is required by post-menopausal women and New Zealand recommendations indicate a level above 1 200 mg may be necessary. The Australian recommendation is to increase the calcium in the basic eating pattern to 1 500 mg per day. Food rich in calcium should be included in the daily food plan. For some women, such as those allergic to milk, a calcium supplement may be recommended.

24
Other nutritional concerns

Sports performance is affected by changes in the lifecycle, age and by the presence of illness or disease. Good nutritional practices play a substantial role in maintaining health and fitness throughout life.

Older athletes

The baseline nutritional needs of a sportsperson over 40 are not substantially different from the requirements of younger sportspeople. Both sportsmen and sportswomen consume more total energy (kilojoules) than their non-athletic or non-active counterparts. Any increase in specific nutrient requirements will generally be met through an increased intake of food.

Advantages of exercise

Exercise considerably slows down the changes in fitness levels that usually occur with advancing age.

Regular exercise appears to have several advantages for older athletes. It improves flexibility and muscle strength and retards bone losses of calcium and other minerals. This is particularly important for women who have passed menopause. Constipation, one of the most frequent medical problems in this age group, is also uncommon in older athletes who exercise regularly. This could result from higher fibre intakes with increased food consumption, or from the exercise increasing the activity of the bowels.

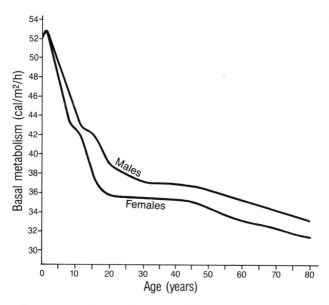

Basal metabolic rates for each sex at different ages.
(Adapted from Guyton, A. C. *Textbook of Medical Physiology.* 5th ed. W. B. Saunders Co., 1976.)

High or raised blood pressure rates seems to be somewhat lower in these athletes compared to non-active people in their age group. This may be associated with lower body weight. There is usually a decrease in muscle mass and an increase in body fat with advancing age. This can be slowed down considerably by continuing regular activity. Weight is also more easily controlled in this way. Several studies indicate blood fat (lipid) levels are kept within a more desirable range in older adults who remain active. All these benefits can reduce the risk of coronary heart disease.

Individuals who do suffer from coronary heart disease should check with their doctor and discuss the exercise programme before commencing. Begin gradually and build up fitness slowly.

Diabetics

Active individuals suffering from diabetes, an inability by the body to process the sugar (glucose) in the blood, will need to make special adaptations when planning their food intake. There are two types of diabetes. One requires insulin to maintain normal blood glucose levels. This is often referred to an insulin-dependent diabetes mellitus

199

(IDDM). Non-insulin-dependent diabetes mellitus (NIDDM) does not generally require insulin, although tablets are sometimes necessary. Food intake and dietary control are essential in the management of both types of diabetes.

The same basic nutritional guidelines for sports performance that apply to the non-diabetic exerciser also apply to the diabetic.

Exercise and diabetes

Regular exercise assists in the management of both types of diabetes. Exercise promotes weight loss and weight control, reduces the effect of carbohydrate ingestion on blood glucose levels and may increase insulin sensitivity. Maintaining activity levels may also decrease the amount of insulin needed.

Exercise and involvement in sports enhances the self-image, improves endurance, and improves blood fat levels for all participants, particularly for the insulin-dependent diabetic. For the non-insulin-dependent diabetic, exercise and dietary control will often control diabetes without the need for medication.

Exercise in a group or with a friend. Do not exercise alone in case you experience a low blood sugar or hypoglycaemic reaction.

Benefits of exercise for diabetics include:

- Improved fitness, muscular strength and endurance.

- Weight control. Exercise uses up kilojoules (or calories) and increases the metabolic rate.

- Lower blood pressure.

- Reduced levels of body fat. Regular exercise and weight loss will result in a loss of body fat stores and an increase in muscle mass.

- A more positive self-image, more energy and the ability to cope more effectively with stress.

There are certain precautions a diabetic must take to reduce the risk of hypoglycaemia while exercising.

Hypoglycaemia is perhaps the major nutritional consideration for the exercising diabetic. It can be a particular problem for the IDDM sufferer because early symptoms may be clouded by hormone responses to exercise. Preparation of pre-exercise snacks or a reduction in insulin doses can prevent hypoglycaemia. This is a personal decision, which should be discussed with the diabetics management team.

For exercise of short duration, such as walking, increase food intake by 1 serving of fruit or bread; around 10–15 g of additional carbohydrate is needed. For moderate intensity exercise lasting about

1 hour, add 20–50 g of carbohydrate foods to your diet. For example, two fruits or a large sandwich. Generally, 1 serving of additional carbohydrate per hour of exercise can be added. However, it must be remembered that these values vary depending on blood glucose control. If levels of blood glucose are high it may not be necessary to include additional servings of carbohydrates. During strenuous exercise monitor your blood glucose levels carefully. Generally, an additional 20–50 g of carbohydrate is adequate.

After unusually strenuous activity, for example during early training or after periods of inactivity, the diabetic sportsperson may experience post-exercise hypoglycaemia. Blood glucose continues to fall as the metabolic rate remains elevated. Attention must also be given to situations in which exercise is performed with high blood sugars caused by insufficient insulin (IDDM) or inadequate control (NIDDM).

Other areas of concern for the active diabetic are care of feet (wear appropriate shoes) and attention to injury to ensure early detection and care. Blood pressure and heart welfare must also be addressed. Aerobic exercise, such as walking and swimming, is beneficial for diabetics. The eyes, kidneys and nerves require specialised care with diabetes. Check with your doctor before commencing an exercise programme.

Additional information for IDDM diabetics

The most important point for the insulin-dependent diabetic is that diabetes should be under good control before starting an exercise programme. Start slowly and gradually increase endurance.

Exercise may cause some changes in blood glucose levels in the the beginning stages of the programme, and these changes can be unpredictable. Careful monitoring of blood glucose levels before, during and after exercise provides a valuable record. Self-testing is the easiest and most convenient method.

An exercising diabetic should be aware of the following factors:

- Exercise lowers blood glucose levels.

- Exercise improves the ability of the body to use glucose.

- The effect of insulin in lowering blood glucose is improved with exercise.

- Note the times when insulin action peaks and decrease the insulin acting during the time of activity.

- Sites for injection require consideration when exercising. Inject insulin in areas not used for the activity. For example, if walking or running inject in the stomach or abdomen rather than the legs.

- The ideal time for exercise is following a meal. Should exercise occur at the time when insulin peaks then plan to eat ahead.

- Additional food may be required because of kilojoules burned during exercise. Eating during exercise is important when activity continues for a long time. This food is an addition to the usual meals and should **not** be subtracted from the eating plan.

- Everyone is different. The effects of exercise on each diabetic vary considerably.

- The type of activity and training schedule influences eating patterns. A sprinter, for example, has different requirements from a marathon runner.

- Testing blood glucose after exercise is important. After exercise, blood glucose levels will continue to decrease. Exercise increases the resting metabolic rate (the amount of energy or kilojoules burned by the body at rest) and blood levels may drop unexpectedly.

Additional information for NIDDM diabetics

For the NIDDM diabetic, exercise will provide many benefits similar to those experienced by the IDDM diabetic. These include:

- Improved control of blood glucose.
- Lowered levels of fat storage.
- Lowered blood cholesterol levels.
- Promotion of weight loss.
- Increased lean muscle mass.
- More effective use of glucose by the muscle.
- Increased sensitivity by the body to insulin or tablets.

The following are additional benefits for the NIDDM diabetic:

- Combining regular exercise with a suitable food plan and weight loss can effectively control NIDDM diabetes.

- The dosage of diabetic medication can be reduced in some cases.

- Blood sugars are more stable during exercise when compared with IDDM diabetes.

The weight loss that occurs while exercising is not a loss of body fat but a loss of body water through sweating. This water must be

202

replaced. Drinking fluids (preferably water) before, during and after exercise is essential to avoid becoming dehydrated.

It is most important that a diabetic's health is fully assessed before exercise commences and as much information as possible provided to enable active diabetics to get maximum benefit and enjoyment from their involvement in their chosen activity or sport.

Athletes with eating disorders

Active people are often very concerned about their body weight. Reports have indicated that athletes are more prone to eating disorders than their non-athletic counterparts. Behaviour patterns which may indicate a destructive eating disorder are: striving for a competitive edge through low body fat and low body weight; images of the body that are extremely distorted; perfectionist attitudes to food; preoccupation with 'the perfect weight'; strict exercise programmes and rigorous dieting; or strict eating patterns.

In attempts to give competitors a winning edge some coaches may encourage weight loss. Extra weight does not help in activities such as gymnastics, figure skating, wrestling, bodybuilding, lightweight rowing, distance running or cycling. However, if excessive amounts of weight are lost, food intake becomes highly controlled, or the athlete fears that his or her weight control is ineffective, anorexia nervosa or bulimic behaviour may occur.

The desire to be a perfect weight has serious consequences for sports performance. Weight loss, often perceived as the major or only goal, is accomplished at the expense of energy levels, adequate nutrition and, in women, maintaining menstruation. The result is a thin, often anaemic, malnourished athlete with little energy left for training.

Anorexia nervosa

Anorexia is often described as self-starvation and, in serious cases, can continue until death. It appears to be more common in women, generally those aged between 12 and 25 years. A significant loss in body weight (over 25 percent of original weight), a body mass index below 17 (healthy weight is 20–25) with a very low percentage of body fat are indicators of this disorder. The women often cease menstruating (amenorrhoea). Accompanying weight loss, sufferers have distorted attitudes towards food and indulge in intense periods of exercise. Even when extremely thin these athletes perceive themselves as fat.

Bulimia or binge eating

Bulimia is harder to detect as weight is usually maintained or can be normal, and the athlete may appear well. Bulimia literally means 'ox hunger'. Periods of uncontrolled eating of large amounts of food are often secretive. Bulimics go to great lengths to conceal their actions. Sometimes the only hint that anything is wrong comes when the athlete involved disappears to the toilet immediately after eating to vomit away the meal just eaten.

Fasting, self-induced vomiting and the abuse of diuretics or laxatives are common methods used to purge the body of food in an attempt to control weight. The vomiting and fluid losses produce several undesirable effects on health including dental decay.

The compulsive eater-exerciser

During the day these athletes eat very little. Both breakfast and lunch are low in fat, sugar and energy. Less than 2.1 MJ have been consumed by the end of the day. However, at night eating becomes uncontrolled. These athletes are starving during the day and bingeing at night. After an evening eating binge the athlete feels that exercise must be performed until all the food eaten has been worked off. Exercise is seen as a form of punishment for the overeating.

Not only is performance impaired by these eating disorders, but there are several health concerns. These include fatigue, fainting, dehydration, electrolyte imbalances (resulting from the use of diet pills and laxative abuse), malnutrition and irregular heartbeat.

Providing help for athletes with eating problems involves a team approach, using a dietitian, doctor and counsellor. The aim of nutritional counselling to help athletes with these types of eating patterns is to replace the destructive pattern with sound practical nutritional practices to get them back to normal eating patterns. Eating disorders are not the problem in themselves but are a symptom of distorted attitudes to body image, unrealistic expectations and emotional problems.

Children and teenagers

Children need special attention as their requirements for growth are different from those of the adult. They have smaller stomachs, require more nutrients and energy-dense foods, and need to develop eating patterns that will promote health in adulthood.

Children require more energy. This energy is used for growth as well as the increased demands of their particular sport or activity. There is some indication that children use more energy than adults. Hence snacks are an important source of additional kilojoules for the active child. Children should be encouraged to eat something before going to school. Breakfast is important and should provide energy (from carbohydrates) and nutrients. It provides a good foundation for the rest of the day. Establishing regular meal patterns is essential.

When considering weight loss for children, increased activity is recommended before restricting energy and food intake. A low-key approach to weight reduction is recommended, focusing on the foods a child can eat rather than on restrictions and limitations.

Active teenagers, such as gymnasts, dancers, wrestlers and light-weight rowers, must find a balance between obtaining adequate energy and nutrients, and maintaining desired body composition for performance. Iron requires special attention. Teenage girls on low-kilojoule weight reduction diets will have lower calcium and zinc intakes. A decrease in sports performance or failure to perform at expected levels may be due to poor nutritional status.

Protein needs

Protein needs are increased during growth. However, there is generally no need for additional supplements of protein as the increase in kilojoules (energy intake) will increase the protein intake. Care is needed with young vegetarians who restrict the intake of red meat and milk in an attempt to control their weight. Obtaining an adequate supply of the essential amino acids is important for growth.

Before puberty, attempts to increase muscle (such as weightlifting and high protein diets) have limited value and can be dangerous. Teenagers wishing to bulk up must be aware that the process is slow, and requires exercise and additional food. The use of anabolic steroids by athletes is no longer limited to adults. Teenagers and children in the United States have reported using these in the belief that the increased muscle and strength will provide a competitive advantage.

Anabolic steroids contain the male sex hormone testosterone (or a synthetic form). These are administered to the body either orally or by injection. Taken in conjunction with an intense exercise programme and a high energy diet anabolic steroids have produced an increase in muscular strength in some individuals.

In children, young adults and women steroid use may be harmful because of the potential of these substances to alter normal body

205

processes. In children and young adults growth may be stunted owing to effects on the bone. Deepening of the voice, acne and changes in the sex organs (lower sperm counts and smaller testicles) are other effects. In women increased facial hair, baldness, irregularities in the menstrual cycle, deepening of the voice and enlargement of the clitoris may result.

Some changes in personality, such as increased aggressive behaviour, have also been reported. Some side-effects are reversible. Others, however, such as the changes (tumors and cancers) to the liver and kidney, are not.

Fluid needs

Children have a proportionally larger surface area and are less effective in sweating and controlling body temperature, when compared with adults. Therefore, fluids are particularly important, especially when exercising in high temperatures. Water intake must be carefully monitored. Do not rely on a child's thirst to replace water losses; if left to their own devices children do not drink sufficient water. Teenagers, as with any person involved in activity, must maintain adequate hydration before, during and after activity, and water is the preferred fluid.

Disabled athletes

Many athletes compete at international level in sports events despite physical handicaps. Nutritional management is part of the care of disabled athletes. Generally, physically disabled athletes should follow the basic principles and recommendations for all sportspeople.

There may, however, be special considerations for individuals. Energy requirements and fluid content require assessment. Particular attention should be given to drug therapy (check for anaemia, increased or decreased appetite, nausea, gastrointestinal disturbances), weight gain and weight loss. Some athletes may experience problems with maintaining muscle tissue. As much as possible a reasonable weight range should be maintained. Some physically disabled athletes will require greater energy, B vitamins and protein intakes, which can be provided using supplements such as Ensure and Polycose. In some cases a multivitamin/mineral supplement may be appropriate.

Weight gain can be a common problem for the disabled, especially in sports requiring a high degree of skill rather than aerobic fitness — for example, shooting and archery. Being overweight further restricts movement. It is important that meals remain enjoyable, but emphasis must be placed on keeping food choices nutrient dense — that is, a high intake of nutrients for fewer kilojoules. Wide changes in weight must be avoided.

A high fibre diet with an increased intake of fluids is recommended to avoid constipation. Flatulence or wind may be a problem for some athletes and requires eating less of the gas-forming fruit and vegetables. These include onions, cauliflower, cabbage and brussels sprouts. If travel is involved it is important to minimise changes in eating patterns and follow a regular pattern.

25
Answers to common questions

Breakfast: Is it important?

Question I frequently miss breakfast. What should I eat to make up for it and when should I eat it?

Answer Not everyone wakes up ready to face a meal. If you find it difficult to eat breakfast try to eat something light. Take in more fuel later in the morning — for example, a glass of fruit juice and yoghurt or perhaps a banana sandwich. Try some fresh melon, fresh fruit or fruit salad, or even a glass of milk and cheese with crackers. Follow this up with a good quality snack at the mid-morning break. Try not to miss meals. If you run late in the morning organise your breakfast the night before. A good quality snack for supper may be appropriate here.

Snacks: Make wholesome choices

Question I often feel like a snack before dinner. What should I eat?

Answer Forget the advertisements that suggest you eat a chocolate-coated candy bar for energy. Select foods with more nutrient impact — for example, fresh fruit, wholegrain sandwiches, low-fat milk, crackers and fruit bars low in sugar. Try banana sandwiches or perhaps a peanut butter sandwich. Remember to allow 2–3 hours for digestion if you have a training session or workout scheduled after work or school.

Plan meals to fit training schedules

Question A triathlete swims at 5.30 in the morning. Should breakfast be eaten before or after the swim? How important is the evening meal?

Answer Breakfast would need to be eaten at 3.30 a.m. to allow for digestion to take place. This is not practical. The evening meal should be high in carbohydrates and you could add a high carbohydrate snack before going to bed. Breakfast can then be eaten later in the morning.

Question A distance runner finds she has difficulty eating food for around 3 hours after a 2-hour run. How much should she eat before she runs and what are some foods that are suitable to eat after her activity?

Answer If running in the afternoon, say after work, then breakfast and lunch should provide the bulk intake of carbohydrate foods and fluids. A slightly larger breakfast and lunch will compensate for a smaller meal in the evening. Fluid will be the most important nutrient. Light fruit drinks, fresh fruit salads, fruit and yoghurt, omelette and salads, sandwiches, pasta with spaghetti sauce and even baked beans on toast are suitable evening meals. A liquid meal replacement may be used occasionally but should not be relied on to provide an adequate nutritional intake. Ensure and Sustagen are two suitable commercial products.

Question A middle distance runner is concerned about her recent loss of appetite. 'I am concerned that I am not getting all the nutrients I need for training. What should I eat and how do I solve this problem?'

Answer A short-term change in appetite can be caused by many factors, such as overtraining, iron deficiency or low glycogen levels. A liquid meal may need to be added during the day to boost energy intake and provide nutrients but it is important that regular food consumption be commenced as soon as possible. Try smaller meals more often. Check that food has not become boring and try to be more creative in the kitchen, which will help to stimulate the appetite.

209

Monitor food intake with changes in exercise levels

Question I am a triathlete who usually exercises regularly. However, during the summer I gained half a stone as I was injured. I had my cholesterol levels checked and discovered they were high. How could this happen?

Answer Exercise helps to keep weight and cholesterol levels low. In fact, one of the benefits of regular exercise is lower cholesterol levels for most people. The weight gain and lower exercise levels, combined with more social eating and drinking over the Christmas season, are largely responsible for the change. Once regular training starts these weight and cholesterol levels should return to normal.

Food before exercise

Question I go to an aerobics class three times a week after school. I tend to eat something just before I go and I generally feel uncomfortable during the class. I usually feel better if I have nothing to eat. Why?

Answer It is not advisable to take vigorous exercise straight after a meal. After eating, the blood supply is diverted to the stomach and digestive system to help with the digestion of the food and the absorption of nutrients. If you exercise immediately after eating the muscle may not receive sufficient blood to work efficiently, or the process of digestion will be slowed as the blood moves from the stomach and digestive system to the muscle. Feeling uncomfortable, sick in the stomach or faint are common in these circumstances.

Exercise and alcohol

Question I enjoy a couple of beers after work and often go to an aerobics class afterwards. Is this harmful and am I getting the best out of my workout?

Answer The effect of alcohol on the nervous system is to impair balance and coordination. Consuming alcohol before exercise may be harmful to performance. In addition to acting as a diuretic, alcohol may decrease the liver's production of glucose, causing low blood sugars. Alcohol does not provide any benefit for exercise or performance. Water is the preferred fluid for most forms of exercise. Wait until the class is finished, then replace fluid loss with water before drinking any form of alcohol.

Fibre: Too much of a good thing

Question   As a runner I usually have no problems with my bowels. As I now eat a very high fibre diet why am I constipated?

Answer   Consuming excessive quantities of fibre can explain these symptoms. Increase fibre intake gradually. Eating large amounts of dietary fibre requires adequate fluid intake to provide full benefit for the bowels because fibre acts with fluid. Increase all fluids, preferably by the addition of water. Anxiety and stress can also alter the activity of the bowels. For some people, excessive intakes of fibre can result in diarrhoea. Everyone has their own individual tolerance level.

Protein powders increase body fat

Question   A boxer asks about bulking up. He has been using protein powders to increase his energy intake. Unfortunately, he has also increased his body fat from 11 percent to 16 percent. 'How did this happen?' he asks.

Answer   An increase in activity, especially strength training, requires a slight increase in protein. The typical food patterns of many New Zealanders provide more than adequate amounts. There is no evidence to suggest that protein powders improve strength, endurance or performance and the additional energy supplied by this excess protein is stored as fat.

In this instance, energy output has not matched energy input and body weight has increased. As the increase in weight was an increase in body fat and not muscle, this explains the change in body fat levels. An additional workload is placed on the kidneys and liver to remove the extra nitrogen from the body. More water is required to dilute and excrete this nitrogen. This may contribute to dehydration. Exercise is an important factor in increasing muscle mass.

Eating out

Question   A cricketer spending a large portion of his time away from home is required to eat out three or four nights a week. He asks how he can maintain a sound nutritional pattern.

Answer   Studies have shown that athletes, and teenagers in particular, perform less well when meals are missed, as this leads to inadequate intakes of energy and other nutrients. By the end of the day several nutrients may have been consumed but they may be below the recommended level. If this occurs over a long period performance can be compromised. When eating takeaway meals, include servings of fresh fruit, fruit juice and salads. Swap french fries for baked potatoes and leave out the salt. Include bean salads and high carbohydrate snacks rather than sweet or fried food. Keep a diary of what has been eaten over a few days and check on the balance of the food choices.

Food for recreational athletes

Question   Is there any special diet for recreational runners?

Answer   Several studies have reported a relationship between diet, exercise and blood lipid levels. Individuals who are active are leaner than their sedentary counterparts. However, there does not appear to be any difference in the general eating pattern of New Zealanders, which remains high in fat. The risk of coronary heart disease is reduced when the person is involved in regular exercise. Exercise assists in blood pressure control, blood fats and weight control. Recreational sportspeople need to follow the same guidelines for their baseline eating patterns as competitive athletes.

Sources of nutrition information

Question   As an aerobics instructor I am often asked questions concerning nutrition. Where can I get reliable information?

Answer   Contact the New Zealand Dietetic Association, your local hospital or dietitians in private practice in your area. Dietitians in New Zealand are registered with the Department of Health, which also has a nutrition section. The National Heart Foundation, New Zealand Nutrition Foundation and Nutrition Society of New Zealand are other sources of information. Addresses are listed in appendix 10.

Appendix 1
Role of vitamins in health and exercise

Abbreviations:

ADI = Adequate daily intake.
This covers 99% of healthy individuals and exceeds nutrient requirements.
It does not account for illness or drug interactions.

MSI = Minimum safe intake.
* Appropriate intake level not identified yet.

RE = Retinol equivalent for vitamin A. 1 μg of B — carotene is equivalent to 0.17 μg of retinol. It takes around 6 micrograms of carotene to produce 1 microgram of vitamin A.

Source: *Recommendations for Selected Nutrient Intake Levels for New Zealanders* (1983).

■ *VITAMIN A*

Retinol (animal source) — carotene (plant source) — fat soluble

Sources	Liver, butter, whole milk, eggs, kidneys, fish oils. Green, yellow, and orange coloured fruit and vegetables: mango, carrots, pumpkin, kumara, spinach, prunes, silverbeet, tomato, broccoli.
Requirement	MSI 600 μg (micrograms) RE ADI 750 μg (micrograms) RE
Function	Essential for growth and development. Prevents night blindness. Keeps skin and the gut maintained in good condition.
Deficiency	If prolonged can lead to nutritional blindness (common in children in developing countries), dry eyes, rough skin, reduced resistance to infection, difficulties with vision in dim light (night blindness).

Excess	Toxic in large amounts, i.e. with excessive supplementation. Loss of appetite, bone pain, dizziness, nausea, vomiting, headaches, muscle fatigue, loss of hair, oedema. Carotenaemia is the orange colour of the skin and palm of the hands. Harmless. Due to excessive intake of carrot juice.
Comment	Mineral oils prevent the absorption of vitamin A. Added to some oils and to margarine. Very little is destroyed in cooking. Stored in the body in the liver.

■ ■ ■

■ VITAMIN B₁

Thiamine — water soluble

Sources	Meat, pork, potatoes, milk, nuts, whole grains, liver, yeast, marmite
Requirement	MSI 0.4 mg ADI 1.2 mg (men) 1.0 mg (women)
Function	Role in the breakdown of carbohydrates to produce energy and in the function of the nervous system and heart.
Deficiency	May occur in people trying to lose weight who remove bread and cereal from the menu. Fatigue, loss of appetite, and irritability occur. Severe deficiency includes disorders of muscles and nerves including the heart (beriberi). Impairs energy production.
Excess	Uncommon. Hypersensitivity described at very low levels of toxicity. Possible interference with absorption of other B vitamins.
Comments	During the refining of cereal foods there are considerable losses. Readily water soluble and unstable to heat. Large losses in cooking. When carbohydrate intake increases there is an increased need for thiamine.

■ ■ ■

■ VITAMIN B₂

Riboflavin — water soluble

Sources	Milk, cheese, liver, yeast, whole grains, cereals, eggs, vegetables.
Requirements	MSI 1.0 mg ADI 1.7 mg
Function	Needed for the production of energy and protein metabolism. Also necessary for growth and healthy skin and eyes.
Deficiency	Deficiency is rare. Changes in the skin, an inflamed tongue, cracks at the corner of the mouth, the eyes become sensitive to light, fatigue.
Excess	No adverse effects have been described.
Comment	Easily destroyed by sunlight. Milk left in the sun for 2-3 hours has 80% of the riboflavin destroyed. Minimal losses in cooking.

■ ■ ■

■ VITAMIN B₃

Niacin — nicotinic acid — water soluble

Sources	Meat, fish, bread, legumes, whole grains, coffee.
Requirements	MSI 5 mg ADI 18 mg
Function	Over 150 enzymes require niacin as a co-factor for the release of energy. Required for a healthy skin. Important for carbohydrate metabolism and fat synthesis.
Deficiency	A mild deficiency can occur with general B vitamin deficiency. Fatigue, skin and mental disturbances are common. A severe deficiency is called pellagra and affects the skin, gut and nervous system.
Excess	Large doses cause dizziness, flushing of the face,

nausea, carbohydrate intolerance and emotional unrest, irregular heartbeat.

Comment   Small amounts can be made from the amino acid tryptophan.
Sometimes promoted as a benefit for schizophrenics.

■ ■ ■

■ VITAMIN B₆

Pyridoxine — water soluble

Sources   Wheatgerm, yeast, liver, whole grains, meat, eggs, soya beans, peanuts, potatoes, fish.

Requirements   MSI   1.25 mg
ADI   2 mg

Function   Needed for amino acid and protein metabolism and has a role in glucose metabolism.
Required for the conversion of the amino acid tryptophan into niacin and for the formation of red blood cells.

Deficiency   Poor growth, anaemia, weakness, irritability, convulsions, loss of appetite, depression and skin lesions.

Excess   Massive doses may produce abnormal liver enzymes and influence nerve function.
Interferes with muscular coordination.

Comment   Easily destroyed by very high temperatures.
Women who take the oral contraceptive pill may have an increased requirement.
An increased need for B₆ with high intakes of protein is possible.

■ ■ ■

■ VITAMIN B₁₂

Cobalamin — an unusual vitamin as it is not made by plants

Sources   Meat, liver, foods of animal origin; fish, eggs, milk, cheese.
Made by some micro-organisms and found in some fermented plant foods, such as tempeh.

Requirements	MSI 1.0 μg ADI 3.0 μg
Function	Responsible for the nervous system and red blood cell development. Also has a role in formation of genetic material.
Deficiency	Pernicious anaemia. Loss of weight, weakness, fatigue, changes in the mental and nervous system, muscular incoordination.
Excess	Possible liver damage.
Comment	Generally not destroyed by cooking except if high temperatures used, such as in frying. Deficiency may occur in strict vegetarians and possibly those taking high doses of vitamin C. When found in food of plant origin it is caused by bacterial contamination.

■ ■ ■

■ BIOTIN

Sources	Liver, kidney, yeast and eggs. Widely distributed in foods.
Requirement	None set. Can be made in the large intestine by gut bacteria.
Function	Role in the metabolism of fats and proteins. Needed for growth and nerve cell function.
Deficiency	Deficiency is very rare. Only occurs if large amounts of raw egg white are eaten (10 eggs per day). Egg white contains avidin which destroys biotin. Loss of appetite, affects growth, nausea, fatigue and depression, muscle ache.
Excess	No adverse effects recognised in humans. Depressed secretion of gastric hydrochloric acid.
Comment	Avidin in egg white is destroyed by the cooking process (see deficiency).

■ ■ ■

■ PANTOTHENIC ACID

Sources	Meat, eggs, whole grains, cereals, legumes, milk, cheese, fish, fruit and vegetables. Most diets adequate in the other B vitamins will contain adequate pantothenic acid.
Requirements	None set.
Function	Needed for the metabolism of fats, carbohydrates and protein.
Deficiency	A deficiency of this vitamin is rare and difficult to produce. Tingling in the hands and feet; may include vomiting, fatigue, cramps and insomnia.
Excess	Diarrhoea, water retention.
Comment	Also synthesised by the gut bacteria but amount needed and significance to humans is unknown.

■ ■ ■

■ FOLIC ACID

Folate or Folacin

Sources	Present in a wide variety of foods such as bread, meat, legumes, and green leaf vegetables.
Requirement	MSI 50 μg ADI 200 μg
Function	Important for formation of genetic material and red blood cell production.
Deficiency	Anaemia (common in pregnant women world wide), reduced endurance.
Excess	Large doses may disguise a vitamin B_{12} deficiency. Possible gastric upset, kidney damage, sleep disturbances.
Comment	Losses in cooking are high as this vitamin is unstable to acid, heat and light. Many drugs interfere with this vitamin: alcohol, diuretics, anticonvulsants, oral contraceptives and tranquillisers.

■ ■ ■

Choline	These are often listed as B vitamins but they

Choline
Inositol
PABA
Lipoic acid
Pangamic acid
(vitamin B$_{15}$)
vitamin B$_{17}$

These are often listed as B vitamins but they are not true vitamins as they are manufactured in the body as needed. They have no known essential nutrient effect for humans.

PABA is para-amino-benzoic acid.
See chapter 16.

■ VITAMIN C

Ascorbic acid — water soluble

Sources
Fresh or frozen fruits and vegetables, parsley, citrus fruit, capsicum, tomato, blackcurrants, pawpaw, bean sprouts, strawberries and cabbage are all rich sources.

Requirement
MSI 10 mg
ADI 60 mg
Extra vitamin C is needed for growing children and women during lactation.

Function
Required for the formation of networks in the body — blood vessels, gums, bones, teeth, collagen, connective tissue, tendons, cartilage.
Also needed for wound healing and the absorption of iron from cereals, fruits and vegetables.
Protects against oxidation.
Resistance to infection.

Deficiency
A lack of this vitamin reduces resistance to infection. Produces tiredness, weakness, poor wound healing, bleeding gums.
Prolonged deficiency, which occurs in alcoholics, elderly living alone, students and people who eat little fresh fruit and vegetables, results in scurvy.
Recovery from training stress may also be slower.

Excess
Megadoses of 2-4 g may cause reproductive failure, reduced B$_{12}$ levels, produce diarrhoea or possibly kidney stones.
A dependency may occur on prolonged large intakes. This may also increase the

requirement for vitamin B_6 and vitamin E. Interferes with copper and iron status.

Comment

One of the most fragile vitamins. Is easily destroyed by cooking. Sensitive to air (O_2), heat, light, metals.

Losses occur due to the action of enzymes caused by bruised, blemished or decaying food, on storage and on thawing.

Some chemicals, such as baking soda, destroy the vitamin.

Cow's milk is a poor source.

■ ■ ■

■ VITAMIN D

Calciferol — fat soluble

Sources

Two major sources:

1. Through the action of the ultraviolet light from the sun on the skin.

2. Food sources include: salmon, herrings, liver, cream, cheese.

Small amounts are found in butter and margarine.

Fish oils are an excellent source if eaten.

Include these foods in a balanced diet as they are not widely distributed in food.

Requirement

MSI *

ADI   10 μg

Function

Responsible for absorption of calcium and phosphorus to be used in formation of bone.

Deficiency

People living indoors and children who are not exposed to sunlight may develop rickets. (Rare in NZ.)

In adults, expecially pregnant women, osteomalacia — softening and bending of the bone — can occur where the skin is not exposed to the sun and diet is deficient in calcium. Can also occur through inadequate calcium metabolism.

Excess

Extreme care is needed with supplements. Safe range of intake very narrow. Toxic levels easily reached.

Loss of appetite, weakness, irritability, vomiting, calcium stones in the lungs and kidneys.

Toxic dose is 45 times the ADI.

Large doses can cause kidney failure.

Comment   Added to margarine and not found in vegetable oils.

In the liver and kidneys vitamin D becomes a hormone to absorb calcium.

A tan or sunburn slows down the formation of vitamin D.

■ ■ ■

■ VITAMIN E

∝-tocopherol — role of this vitamin not fully understood — fat soluble

Sources   Rich sources: vegetable oils, sunflower, sesame, wheatgerm, seeds.

Good sources: whole grains, eggs, butter.

Poor sources: meat, fruit, vegetables, refined cereals.

Widely distributed in the diet.

Requirements   MSI   3.5 mg

ADI   13.5 mg (men)   10.0 mg (women)

Function   Antioxidant and provides stability to structure of membranes.

Protects fats and vitamin A from oxidation.

Deficiency   Occurs with fat malabsorption.

Seen as premature destruction of red blood cells (haemolytic anaemia) in newborn babies.

Infant formulas in NZ contain vitamin E supplement.

Reduced resistance to tissue oxidation.

Excess   Harmful doses (above 800 mg/day) have caused muscle weakness, disturbances of the gut and of reproduction.

Vitamin C deficiency may result from an excessive intake.

Becomes less efficient as the intake is increased.

Interferes with the absorption of vitamins A and K.
Depression, fatigue.

Comment
Stored in the fat (adipose) tissue.
Much is destroyed by deep frying.
Many false claims made about vitamin E, but scientific research has failed to prove any of the claims. These include that it cures heart disease, dry skin, acne, infertility, warts, diabetes and cancer.

■ ■ ■

■ VITAMIN K

Fat soluble

Sources
1. Food sources include: green-leaf vegetables like silverbeet, soya beans, eggs and liver.
2. Bacteria of the gut also produce some of this vitamin.

Requirement
Very small amount required through food as it is also manufactured by the gut bacteria.

Function
Essential for formation of blood clots (for prothrombin).

Deficiency
A deficiency can lead to excessive bleeding and haemorrhages.
This can also occur with overdoses of anticoagulants or with fat malabsorption.
Impaired blood clotting.
Rare.

Excess
May induce a deficiency of vitamin E. May interfere with normal blood clotting. Anaemia in infants.

Comment
Fat soluble so little lost due to cooking.
Not absorbed from food if a mineral oil is taken.
Destroyed by long exposure to sunlight.

■ ■ ■

Appendix 2
Role of minerals in health and exercise

Abbreviations:
ADI = Adequate daily intake
MSI = Minimum safe intake

■ CALCIUM

Sources	Milk (all forms), cheese, yoghurt, fish with edible bones (salmon, sardines), green-leaf vegetables, tofu. Some in whole grains and nuts. Eggs, butter, cream and potato are poor sources.
Requirement	MSI 400 mg ADI 600 mg
Function	Acts with phosphorus in the structure of bone and teeth. Role in blood clotting, transmission of nerve impulses, growth, muscle contraction, relaxation, muscle and liver glycogen.
Deficiency	Muscle cramp. With a lack of calcium, phosphorus or vitamin D rickets develops in children (rare in NZ). Osteoporosis caused by low calcium plus hormonal factors (more common in women after menopause).
Excess	Possible kidney stones, muscle and bone changes.
Comment	99% of calcium found in bones and teeth. Stored in bones to maintain blood levels and cells.

High protein intakes can cause losses in the urine.
Excess fibre can bind the mineral making it unavailable for absorption.

■ ■ ■

■ CHLORINE

Sources	Table salt, sea salt, rock salt.
Requirement	No ADI recommended.
Function	Responsible for electrolyte and fluid balance in the body
Deficiency	Reduced appetite, possible muscle cramp and mental apathy.
Excess	Vomiting.
Comment	Some also supplied in the water supply.

■ ■ ■

■ MAGNESIUM

Sources

Green-leaf vegetables are good source.
Meat, fish, fruit, cereals, nuts and vegetables are moderate sources.

Requirement

MSI	Men	200 mg
ADI	Men	350 mg
MSI	Women	200 mg
ADI	Women	300 mg

Function

Role in protein synthesis and muscle contraction important for reactions in the production of energy, body temperature regulation, bone and calcium.

Deficiency

Occurs after a long absence of normal food intake (alcoholics).
Causes disturbances in heart, weakness and growth failure, diarrhoea.

Excess

Possible diarrhoea.

Comment

Eating a wide selection of foods, especially vegetables, provides adequate magnesium.

■ ■ ■

■ PHOSPHORUS

Sources	Milk, cheese and yoghurt are good sources. Moderate amounts in meat, fish and cereals.
Requirement	Related to calcium intake. No problems in obtaining an adequate supply.
Function	Works with calcium in the structure of bone and teeth. Involved in energy release as ATP (adenosine triphosphate).
Deficiency	When dietary calcium is low, calcium from the skeleton is transferred to the blood and rickets results.
Excess	Erosion of jaw (rare).
Comment	Soft drinks and soda drinks, high in this mineral, influence levels and absorption of calcium.

■ ■ ■

■ POTASSIUM

Sources	Dried fruit is excellent food source. Moderate amounts in meat, fish, milk, vegetables, eggs and cereals.
Requirement	No ADI recommended.
Function	Involved in muscle function and regulation and maintains body fluids, including acid base balance of blood.
Deficiency	Problems occur when normal eating stops or diuretics are used, affecting heart muscle.
Excess	Muscular weakness. Excessive storage of potassium in the body can cause cardiac arrest and death.
Comment	Changes in this mineral produce heart irregularities. Works inside the cell and regulated by the kidney.

■ ■ ■

■ SODIUM

Sources	Seafood, processed foods, bread, canned foods with salt, soya sauce, yeast spreads and table salt are all high sources.

Requirement	Moderate intake is recommended.
Function	An important mineral. Works with potassium in maintaining cell fluid balance.
Deficiency	Apathy, vomiting, distress. Occurs with excessive sweating, working in hot weather, exercise in hot climates. Replace fluids immediately.
Excess	Easily added to foods. Excess occurs with disease of kidney, water retention, use of salt tablets. High blood pressure in susceptible people, dehydration, cramp.
Comment	A common electrolyte working outside the cell. Excess is normally excreted by the kidney in the urine.

■ ■ ■

■ IRON

Sources	Rich sources of iron include liver, kidney and dried apricots. Moderate sources include meat, egg, vegetables, wholegrain cereals and dried beans.
Requirement	MSI Men 5 mg ADI Men 10 mg MSI Women 5 mg ADI Women 12 mg
Function	Essential for the transport and utilisation of oxygen and important for many enzymes. Required for the formation of haemoglobin.
Deficiency	Anaemia. Reduces resistance to infection. Reduces the capacity to exercise by reducing oxygen flow to the muscle.
Excess	Excess is rare but can cause liver damage.
Comment	Only around 10% iron is absorbed from food. Absorption increased with vitamin C and decreased with phytic acid.

■ ■ ■

■ COPPER

Sources	Liver, brains and kidneys are all excellent sources of copper. More common sources include: eggs, cereals, meat and vegetables.
Requirement	MSI 1.5 mg ADI 2.5 mg
Function	Part of many enzymes, required for normal growth, and has a role in the formation of haemoglobin.
Deficiency	Anaemia
Excess	Wilson's disease (rare).

■ ■ ■

■ ZINC

Sources	Zinc is found in oysters, gelatine and wheat-germ in reasonable amounts. More common sources are: meat, egg, liver, wholegrain cereals and milk.
Requirement	MSI 8 mg ADI 15 mg
Function	Important for wound healing and growth. Part of many enzymes and assists with protein and carbohydrate metabolism.
Deficiency	Delays growth, depresses appetite and delays wound healing. Possible decrease in the senses of taste and smell.
Excess	Can cause vomiting and fever. Decreases the absorption of other minerals. Increases cholesterol levels.
Comment	Deficiency often associated with alcoholism.

■ ■ ■

■ SELENIUM

Sources	Seafoods, fish, kidney and liver are all good sources.
Requirement	No ADI established.

Function	Acts as an antioxidant to help protect cells from oxidation. Possible role with vitamin E.
Deficiency	Possible effect on heart.
Excess	Gastrointestinal disorders.
Comment	Although the NZ soil is low in this element, a deficiency appears unlikely.

■ ■ ■

■ CHROMIUM

Sources	Brewer's yeast is an excellent food source. More common sources include wholegrain cereals and liver.
Requirement	No ADI established.
Function	Helps control glucose metabolism with insulin and is involved in carbohydrate and fat metabolism.
Deficiency	Impaired ability to metabolise glucose.
Excess	Environmental and occupational exposure can cause skin and kidney damage.

■ ■ ■

■ CADMIUM, NICKEL, TIN, SILICON, LEAD, MERCURY

Sources	Most animal and plant foods contain these minerals. It is unlikely to find the general diet deficient in these elements.
Requirement	No ADI established.
Function	Various enzymes and body tissues.
Deficiency	Deficiency is unlikely.
Excess	Lead accumulating in the body causes anaemia and damage to the brain and kidneys. Usually caused by occupational exposures.
Comment	Some concern about mercury levels in people who eat large amounts of fish.

■ ■ ■

■ *IODINE*

Sources	Seafoods are a rich source. Iodised salt (40–80 ppm).
Requirement	Use of iodised salt provides sufficient. MSI 100 μg ADI 200 μg
Function	Required by the thyroid gland to produce the hormone which controls basal metabolic rate: thyroxine.
Deficiency	Goitre: enlarged thyroid gland.
Excess	Excess may depress the action of the thyroid gland.
Comment	Iodine from kelp (seaweed) will not promote weight reduction. Iodine is essential for normal metabolism and will not increase metabolism.

■ ■ ■

■ *FLUORIDE*

Sources	Tea and water.
Requirement	MSI 1 mg ADI 3 mg
Function	Prevents tooth decay. Important for the maintenance and growth of bone.
Deficiency	High frequency of dental caries (tooth decay).
Excess	Mottling of the teeth (found where naturally high levels of fluoride are present).

■ ■ ■

Appendix 3
Food choice exchange lists

Food can be divided into a number of groups depending on the nutrient each food provides. The major food groups are: meat, fish, poultry and legumes; milk and milk products; bread and cereals; fruit and vegetables; fats, sweets and alcohol. Foods belonging to each group can be divided further according to their energy (calorie) content. Each serving listed is one choice which can be exchanged for another food from the same group.

Meat, fish, poultry and legumes
Choose lean meat, skim off all fat and take care with serving sizes.

Beef:	lean roasted	1 slice	Fish:	Crabmeat†	½ cup
	lean minced	½ cup		Crayfish †	½ cup
	stewed/ casseroled	½ cup		Mussels	½ cup
Oxtail		½ cup		Salmon*	½ cup
Veal/Pork		1 slice		Tuna*	½ cup
Ham*		1 slice		Oysters†	½ cup
Bacon*					
Lamb		1 slice		Scallops†	½ cup
Mutton					
Chicken	(no skin)	1 leg		Shellfish†	½ cup
Duck/Turkey		½ cup		Snapper	½ cup
Kidney		½ cup		Egg	1
Liver†					
Tripe		½ cup		Baked beans	½ cup
Brains†					
Sweetbreads		½ cup		Legumes	½ cup

*Foods high in salt
†Foods high in cholesterol

Note 1:
One serving of pastry (as in meat pies), baked beans or legumes counts as an additional serving of bread, cereal (rice), fruit or vegetable (pumpkin) in addition to the meat choice.

Note 2:
Foods with a high fat content, which may be eaten in small quantities occasionally, include: salami*, luncheon sausage*, sausages*, sardines (use water-processed varieties), and pastry* (meat pies and savouries).

■ ■ ■

Milk, cheese and milk products

Choose the lower fat varieties or smaller servings of foods with a higher fat content.

Milk:	skim, 300 ml	Cheese:	cottage, 75 g
	trim, 300 ml		processed, 2 slices
	homogenised, 220 ml		cheddar*, 50 g
	whole, 180 ml		brie/camembert
	evaporated, 100 ml		edam/gouda
	condensed,		mozzarella ricotta
Yoghurt:	slimmers, 200 g	Ice cream:	full cream
	natural, 150 g		soya based
	fruit, 100 g	Tofu:	1 small scoop

*Foods high in salt
Note: One serving of ice cream or yoghurt counts as one additional serving of bread, cereal (rice), fruit or vegetable (kumara).

■ ■ ■

Bread and cereals

Wholegrain products or varieties are preferable.

½ thick bread	½ cup rice	Cereals (½ cup):
1 thin bread	½ cup noodles	All Bran
½ bun	½ cup macaroni	cornflakes
½ roll	½ cup spaghetti	Kornies
3 crackers*	½ cup baked beans	muesli
2 crackers (large)	½ cup rice flakes	oatbran
2 biscuits (plain)	¼ cup oats	porridge
1 biscuit (sweet)	2 tbsp ground rice	wheatgerm
1 muffin	½ cake	Puffed Wheat
½ scone	¼ pizza (small base)	Rice Bubbles
1 cup soup*	1 pancake	Ricies
2 tbsp white sauce*	1 tortilla*	Weetbix
¹/3 cup pastry*†	2 tbsp corn chips*	
2 tbsp gravy*†	1 pita bread (small)	
2 tbsp flour	½ pita bread (large)	
2 tbsp breadcrumbs		

*Foods high in salt
†Foods high in cholesterol

■ ■ ■

Fruit and vegetables

Foods from this food group should be raw, unpeeled, microwaved, or lightly steamed where possible. One serving from this group can be exchanged for one serving from the bread and cereal food group. One serving of stewed fruit equals half a cup without sweetening.

Fruit

1 apple	1 grapefruit	1 peach
2 apricots (fresh)	¹/3 cup grapefruit juice	1 pear
2 apricots (dried)	½ cup grapes	¼ cup chutney
¼ avocado	½ cup guava	2 tbsp pickle
½ banana	1 kiwifruit	½ cup pineapple
½ cup blackberries	2 mandarins	2 plums
½ cup blueberries	½ cup mango	3 prunes (small)
½ cup boysenberries	6 olives	½ cup raspberries,
½ cup cherries	1 orange	½ cup strawberries
½ cup cranberries	½ cup papaya	¼ cup dried fruit
3 dates	6 passionfruit	1 tangelo
2 figs	½ cup pawpaw	½ cup fruit juice
2 feijoas	½ cup melon	(dilute 50/50)

Vegetables

½ cup beetroot	½ cup kumara	½ cup sweetcorn
½ cup breadfruit	½ cup mixed veges	½ cup taro
½ cup broad beans	½ cup parsnip	½ cup turnip
½ cup butternut	½ cup peas	3 yams
½ cup cassava	½ cup potato	1 cup carrots
½ cup coconut	½ cup pumpkin	1 cup vegetable
1 sml corn cob	½ cup squash	juice (except tomato)

See 'Foods allowed freely' table for additional fruit and vegetables.

■ ■ ■

Fats, sweets and alcohol

The daily fat allowance is 2 teaspoons.

1 tsp butter*/marg	1 tsp cream*	1 tsp sugar:
1 tsp dripping*	1 tsp cream cheese*	white
1 tsp Chefade*	1 tsp sour cream*	raw
1 tsp lard*	1 tsp salad dressing*	brown
1 tsp oil:	1 tsp mayonnaise*	1 tsp jam
peanut	1 tsp tartare sauce*	1 tsp honey
sunflower	1 x chocolate*	1 tsp syrup:
soya bean	½ pkt chips*	maple
olive	1 cup jelly	golden
safflower	2 tbsp coconut	pancake
coconut*	1 cup soft drink	2 candy/sweets
2 tsp nuts:	4 tsp seeds:	1 tsp peanut butter
walnuts	pumpkin	
almonds	sesame	
peanuts	sunflower	

Alcohol:
  beer, 1 small glass/bottle/can
  wine, 1 glass dry white with soda water
  spirits, 1 small nip whisky/gin/vodka

*Foods high in cholesterol

■ ■ ■

Foods allowed freely

Vegetables

Artichokes	Celery	Radishes
Asparagus	Courgettes	Red peppers
Bamboo shoots	Cucumber	Silverbeet
Butter beans	Egg plant	Spinach
Beans, French	Green pepper	Sprouts, alfalfa
Beans, runner	Kamokamo	Sprouts, mung bean
Broccoli	Leeks	Swede
Brussels sprouts	Lettuce	Sugarsnap peas
Cabbage, green	Marrow	Tomato
Cabbage, red	Mushroom	Turnip
Carrot	Onion	Watercress
Cauliflower	Puha	

Fruit

Gooseberries	Lemon	Lime
Honeydew melon	NZ guava	Rhubarb
Cantaloup	Passionfruit (2)	Tamarillo (2)
Watermelon (1 slice)		

Other

Tea	Herbs	Salt*
Herbal tea	Spices	Clear soup*
Coffee	Garlic	Trim soup*
Lemon juice	Essences	Vegemite*
Lime juice	Mustard	Marmite*
Tomato juice	Curry powder	Soya sauce*
Low energy drinks	BBQ sauce	Worcestershire sauce*
Diet soda	Tomato sauce	Gelatin
Mineral water	Pepper	Low cal jelly
Slim tonic water	Vinegar	Popcorn (2 tbsp)
Bran flakes (2 tbsp)	Low cal dressing (2 tsp)	

* Foods high in salt

■ ■ ■

Appendix 4

Average energy intakes

The following table shows average energy intakes for groups of healthy individuals at normal activity levels. (Information supplied by the Nutrition Advisory Committee, 1983.)

Infants:	MJ/day	Cal/day
0–3 mth	0.48/kg	115/kg
3–12 mth	0.42/kg	100/kg
1–3 yr	6.0	1 435
3–5 yr	6.5	1 550
6–8 yr	8.0	1 910
Boys:		
9–11 yr	9.5	2 270
12–14 yr	11.0	2 630
15–17 yr	12.0	2 870
Girls:		
9–11 yr	8.5	2 030
12–14 yr	9.0	2 150
15–17 yr	9.0	2 150
Adult males	11.0	2 630
Adult females	8.5	2 030
During pregnancy	10.0	2 390
During lactation	11.5	2 750

■ ■ ■

Appendix 5
Recommended intakes of selected foods

MSI = minimum safe intake;   ADI = adequate daily intake;   RE = Retinol equivalents for vitamin A;   Vitamin E as α — tocopherol.

Notes: **The minimum safe intake** (MSI) is the level below which there is a substantial likelihood of adverse health consequences.
The adequate daily intake (ADI) is a level of intake which should be at least sufficient for the great majority of healthy people.

	Protein (g)		Vit A (µgRE)		Vit D (µg)		Vit E (mg)		Thiamin (mg)		Riboflavin (mg)	
	MSI	ADI	MSI	ADI	MSI	ADI	MSI	ADI	MSI	ADI	MSI	ADI
Infants												
0-6mths	1.8 g/kg	2.2 g/kg	10 µg/kg	300	2.5	7.5	1.5	3	0.1	0.2	0.3	0.4
1-12mths	1.4 g/kg	1.7 g/kg	10 µg/kg	450	3.5	5	1.5	4	0.3	0.4	0.3	0.4
Children												
1-3 yrs	12	35		300		10		5		0.6		0.7
3-5 yrs	16	45		300		10		6		0.7		0.9
6-8 yrs	20	50		400		10		7		0.8		1.0
Boys												
9-11 yrs	25	57		575		10		10		0.9		1.2
12-14 yrs	30	66		725		10		10		1.1		1.4
15-17 yrs	28	72		750		10	3.5	13.5		1.2		1.7
Girls												
9-11 yrs	23	51		575		10		10		0.8		1.2
12-14 yrs	26	53		725		10		10		0.9		1.4
15-17 yrs	29	53		750		10	3.5	10		0.9		1.7
Adult men	35	65	600	750		10	3.5	13.5	0.4	1.2	1.0	1.7
Adult women	35	50	600	750		10	3.5	10	0.4	1.0	1.0	1.7
Pregnancy		60		750		10		10		1.1		2.5
Lactation		70		1200		10		10		1.2		2.5

	Niacin (mg)		Pyridoxine (mg)		Folate (μg)		Iron (mg)		Calcium	
	MSI	ADI	MSI	ADI	MSI	ADI	MSI	ADI	MSI	ADI
Infants										
0-6 mths	2	5	0.1	0.4	20	50		6	300	600
6-12 mths	3	5	0.2	0.4	20	50		6	300	600
Children										
1-3 yrs		8		0.6		100		7	300	600
3-5 yrs		10		0.9		100		10	200	600
6-8 yrs		11		1.2		200		10	200	600
Boys										
9-11 yrs		14		1.2		200		12	300	700
12-14 yrs		16		1.6		200		12	400	800
15-17 yrs		19		2.0		200		12	400	800
Girls										
9-11 yrs		14		1.2		200		12	400	800
12-14 yrs		16		1.6		200		12	400	800
15-17 yrs		19		2.0		200		12	400	800
Adult men	5	18	1.25	2.0	50	200	5	10	400	600
Adult women	5	18	1.25	2.0	50	200	5	12	400	600
During pregnancy		18		2.5	250	500	12	15	1000	1200
During lactation		21		2.5		400	10	13	1000	1200

	B12 (µg)		Vit C (mg)		Copper (mg)		Zinc (mg)		Iodine (µg)		Fluoride (mg)	
	MSI	ADI	MSI	ADI	MSI	ADI	MSI	ADI	MSI	ADI	MSI	ADI
					(µg)							
Infants												
0-6 mths		0.3	5	20	20/kg	60/kg		3		35	0.1	0.5
6-12 yrs		0.3	5	20	20/kg	60/kg		3		35	0.1	0.5
Children					(mg)							
1-3 yrs		0.3		25		1.2		5		45		1
3-5 yrs		1.5		30		1.5		8		60		1
6-8 yrs		2.0		30		2.1		10		80		1
Boys												
9-11 yrs		3.0		35		2.5		15		100		1.5
12-14 yrs		3.0		50		2.5		15		150		2
15-17 yrs		3.0		60		2.5		15		200	1	3
Girls												
9-11 yrs		3.0		35		2.5		15		100		1.5
12-14 yrs		3.0		45		2.5		15		150		2
15-17 yrs		3.0		60		2.5		15		200	1	3
Adult men	1.0	3.0	10	60	1.5	2.5	8	15	100	200	1	3
Adult women	1.0	3.0	10	60	1.5	2.5	8	15	100	200	1	3
During pregnancy	1.6	4.0		70		3.0		20	100	200	1	3
During lactation	1.5	4.0		70		2.5		25	100	200	1	3

Appendix 6
Guidelines for using supplements

1. A supplement should contain no more than 100 percent of the adequate daily intake (ADI). Products that contain less are preferred.

2. A multivitamin and mineral preparation is more suitable than a single nutrient.

3. Read the labels carefully and compare with the ADI recommendations. Make sure you know what is in the supplement and how much of each ingredient it contains.

4. Avoid supplements with non-nutritive additives. These include herbs, pangamic acid and garlic. These substances have no nutritional benefit and add to the cost. They are easily identified as there is no ADI listed on the label.

5. High potency and stress formulas or therapeutic doses of supplements are not recommended. These may contain vitamins and minerals at almost toxic levels.

6. Natural or organic supplements are more expensive and no more beneficial than regular supplements. The body is unable to detect the difference between natural and synthetic varieties.

7. No supplement will make up for a poor diet or inadequate eating patterns. Vitamin and mineral supplements do not contain protein, carbohydrate or fat, which are essential for sports performance.

8. Many nutrients, such as iron, are absorbed more effectively from foods than from pills.

9. Consult a dietitian or doctor before embarking on self-medication with supplements.

10. The best insurance is to eat a wide selection of food.

Appendix 7

Additives permitted in manufactured foods

(Information adapted from data supplied by the Department of Health pamphlet code 4145.) A full list of food additives is available from district offices of the Department of Health.

Preservatives Code no.	Additive	Colours Code no.	Additive
200	Sorbic acid	102	Tartrazine
210	Benzoic acid	110	Sunset yellow
223	Sodium metabisulphite	120	Cochineal
250	Sodium nitrite	123	Amaranth
251	Sodium nitrate	132	Indigotine
260	Acetic acid	133	Brilliant blue
261	Potassium acetate	140	Chlorophyll
262	Sodium acetate	142	Green S
270	Lactic acid	150	Caramel
280	Propionic acid	160	Beta carotene
290	Carbon dioxide		
296	Mulic acid		
300	Ascorbic acid		

■ ■ ■

Emulsifiers & thickeners

Code no.	Additive
322	Lecithin
330	Citric acid
339	Sodium phosphate
400	Alginic acid
406	Agar
410	Locust bean gum
412	Guar gum
440	Pectin

Antioxidants

Code no.	Additive
300	Ascorbic acid
306	Tocopherol
310	Propyl gallate
320	BHA
321	BHT
330	Citric acid
334	Tartaric acid

Other common code numbers

Code no.	Additive	Function
420	Sorbitol	Sweetener
621	MSG	Flavour enhancer
627	Sodium guanylate	Flavour enhancer

Note: Some additives perform more than one function.

Appendix 8
Banned substances

Since the early 1960s there has been an increasing use of performance-enhancing drugs in sport. As new products to improve performance have emerged, the International Olympic Committee has moved to outlaw their use. With more and more money at stake for competitors the incentive to use banned substances has increased. Since the Seoul Olympics, where Canadian athlete Ben Johnson was caught using stenozolol (an anabolic steroid), there has been high international exposure of the problem and efforts at international level to control it.

The banned substances fall into the following groups: stimulants; narcotics; anabolic steroids; beta-blockers; and diuretics. As well as these classes, there are the Growth Hormone and Human Chorionic Gonadotropin — naturally occurring hormones used to achieve an anabolic effect. Also banned is 'blood doping', the procedure whereby blood is taken from the competitor six weeks in advance of a major event, then, when his or her body has regenerated new red blood cells to replace those lost, the extracted blood is reinfused. The athlete thus achieves an elevated haemoglobin and, presumably, an increased oxygen-carrying capacity.

In recent years masking agents have been used to hide the use of banned drugs. These have included diuretics (now banned) and probenaid (a drug used to treat gout), which blocks the excretion of steroids in the urine.

Perhaps the major problem for the athlete is to avoid inadvertently taking a banned substance. Obviously an elite athlete wouldn't use morphine (banned as a narcotic analgesic), but he or she might use Panadeine, which contains codeine. Unfortunately codeine breakdown products resemble narcotic breakdown products, and Panadeine is thus a banned substance. Similarly ephidrine is a banned

243

stimulant, but nasal sprays sold in New Zealand, such as Neo-Synophrine, contain pseudo ephidrine (a related compound) and are therefore also banned. Other nasal sprays such as Otrivine and Drixine are perfectly legal. There are also many cough mixtures which contain ephidrine-related substances, so the utmost caution needs to be exercised so as not to inadvertently take a banned substance. Vicks Formula 44, a cough medicine containing Dextromethorphan, is legal.

It is clear, therefore, that the sports competitor should not use preparations without being fully aware of their contents, nor should he or she take anything prescribed by a doctor without being convinced it contains no banned substances.

Doping classes
A. Stimulants
B. Narcotics
C. Anabolic steroids
D. Beta-blockers
E. Diuretics

Doping methods
A. Blood doping
B. Pharmacological, chemical and physical manipulation

Classes of drugs subject to certain restrictions
A. Alcohol
B. Local anaesthetics
C. Corticosteroids

In New Zealand we have embarked on a random drug-testing programme, which involves the taking of urine specimens on a random basis outside the competition context. All sports affiliated to the New Zealand Olympic and Commonwealth Games Association are involved, and the sports participants know they may be asked, at 48 hours' notice, to provide a specimen. These specimens are sent to an IOC-accredited laboratory for analysis.

Systems such as New Zealand's have in the past fallen into disrepute because of rumours of competitors being warned in advance, being let off after a positive sample, or being assured they wouldn't be picked for testing at a big meeting. If our programme is to be successful it must be seen to be beyond reproach and completely impartial. While the system is seen to be fair we can expect to gain the respect of the athletes and they will continue to endorse the programme.

In summary, while the problem of illegal sports drug-taking is relatively small in New Zealand it is to our credit that the authorities have moved to control the increase in usage. While it could have an adverse effect on our medal count, as countries with an effective random testing programme have found, it can only improve our prestige in the sporting world.

Dr Tony Edwards
Chairman of the drugs in sport subcommittee,
New Zealand Federation of Sports Medicine.

Appendix 9
Sports drinks

Comparison of sports drinks per cup (250 ml):

Drink	Energy source	Energy kJ	CHO %	Na mg	K mg
Exceed fluid replacement	Glucose polymers	293	7	50	45
Apple juice	Fructose } Glucose	440	11	8	368
Orange juice	Fructose } Sucrose Glucose	450	11	2	408
Cola drinks	Fructose } Sucrose	435	10	10	2.5
Lucozade	Glucose	773	18	65–75	2–4
Replace	Glucose } Maltodextrins	237	6	43	31
Sustalyte	Dextrose	303	8	253	429
Gatorade	Sucrose } Glucose	209	6	110	25
Shanklee Sport	Glucose polymer } Fructose Dextrose	225	6	63	38

■ ■ ■

Appendix 10
Sources of nutrition information

NZ Dietetic Association
P O Box 5065   WELLINGTON

Consumer and Applied Science Department
University of Otago
P O Box 56   DUNEDIN

NZ Nutrition Foundation
P O Box 31185   Milford   AUCKLAND

Department of Health
P O Box 5013   WELLINGTON

Nutrition Society of New Zealand
Massey University
Private Bag   PALMERSTON NORTH

National Heart Foundation
P O Box 17128   Greenlane   AUCKLAND

DSIR
Department of Scientific and Industrial Research
Science Information Publishing Centre
P O Box 9741   WELLINGTON

Dairy Advisory Bureau
P O Box 9890   Newmarket   AUCKLAND

Bibliography

Clark, Nancy. *The Athlete's Kitchen.* New York, 1981.

Coleman, Ellen. *Eating for Endurance.* Palo Alto, California, 1988.

Eisenman, P., and Johnson, D. *The Coach's Guide to Nutrition and Weight Control.* Champaign, Illinois, 1982.

Fox, Edward, and Matthews, Donald. *The Physiological Basis of Physical Education and Athletics.* Philadelphia, 1981.

Gillies, M., and Swindells, Y. *Today's Food — Tomorrow's Health.* University of Otago, Dunedin, 1986.

Inge, Karen, and Brukner, Peter. *Food for Sport.* Melbourne, 1986.

Katch, F., and McArdle, W. *Nutrition, Weight Control and Exercise.* Philadelphia, 1983.

Marcus, Jacqueline (ed). *Sports Nutrition: A Guide for the Professional Working with Active People.* Chicago, 1986.

McArdle, William; Katch, Frank; and Katch, Victor. *Exercise Physiology: Energy, Nutrition and Human Performance.* Philadelphia, 1981.

Rafoth, Richard. *Bicycling Fuel: Nutrition for Bicycle Riders.* Mill Valley, California, 1988.

Smith, Nathan. *Food for Sport.* California, 1976.

Williams, Melvin. *Nutritional Aspects of Human Physical and Athletic Performance.* Second edition. Springfield, Illinois, 1985.